Test Question Logic

(TQLogic™) for the NCLEX-RN Exam

SIXTH EDITION

PATRICIA A. HOEFLER, M.S.N., R.N.

AUTHOR

meds
PUBLISHING

MEDICAL EDUCATION DEVELOPMENT SERVICES

4000 BLACKBURN LANE, SUITE 260

BURTONSVILLE, MARYLAND 20866

www.medspub.com

Editor: Mark Williams-Abrams

SIXTH EDITION 2004

Copies of this book may be obtained from:
MEDICAL EDUCATION DEVELOPMENT SERVICES
4000 Blackburn Lane, Suite 260
Burtonsville, Maryland 20866
www.medspub.com

ISBN: 1-56533-505-8
Printed in the United States of America.

Table of Contents

Introduction

WHY A BOOK ON PROBLEM-SOLVING AND TEST-TAKING FOR NURSING EXAMS?

The purpose of this book is to help you master the test-taking skills needed to do well on your nursing course exams and, ultimately, on the NCLEX-RN Exam and other professional nursing examinations.

> ## The material in this book is important because test taking has become an essential professional skill.

The problem-solving and analytical skills discussed in this book are useful throughout nursing school, for the NCLEX-RN Exam, and throughout your nursing career.

Test taking is not presently taught in most nursing programs. This book was written to fill a gap in the standard nursing curriculum. Written by a nurse educator with well over two decades of grass roots experience in presenting NCLEX-RN Exam review courses and test-taking seminars across the U.S. and Canada, *Test Question Logic (TQLogic™) for the NCLEX-RN Exam* addresses your needs as a nursing student and NCLEX-RN Exam candidate, and its methods respect the nursing profession. The test-taking guidelines and strategies in this book will help you to look at test questions from a different perspective. With the training and practice you'll find in this book, you can become more analytical and a better problem solver!

Since you began taking nursing courses, have you heard yourself making the following comments?

"I do very well clinically, but I do poorly on the nursing exams. Why are the questions so hard?"

"I get excellent grades clinically, but the scores on my nursing exams decrease my overall grade in nursing."

"I study very hard, but my nursing exam grades do not show it. The test questions are so confusing. Why don't the instructors learn to write clearer test questions so that I can answer them?"

The NCLEX-RN Exam, of course, presents additional challenges. If you are getting ready to take the NCLEX-RN Exam, are you nervous about preparing for it? Are you and your fellow students asking yourselves:

"How can I possibly review all my nursing content before the exam?"

"What's the computerized NCLEX-RN like? And how do I know that I will get a fair selection of questions with the new computerized adaptive testing?"

"Is there any way to practice answering NCLEX-RN-type questions before I take the exam?"

If you find nursing exams difficult, you are not alone! Like many other nursing students, you probably find taking multiple choice nursing examinations a stressful experience. But nursing exams—even the NCLEX-RN—don't have to be quite so stressful or worrisome!

Research has demonstrated that regardless of how similar the educational background and training of any two students may be, the test-wise candidate will score higher, on average, than the less skilled test taker every time.

This is also true for nursing exams. Learning how to effectively prepare for an exam and improving your test-taking skills will **decrease test-taking anxiety** and enable you to **make the most of your nursing knowledge**. This book is dedicated to helping you do just that. With *Test Question Logic (TQLogic™) for the NCLEX-RN Exam,* you can improve your score on nursing exams and on the NCLEX-RN!

WHY ARE NURSING EXAMS SO DIFFICULT?

Today's nursing students are highly motivated, very capable students. Before entering nursing school, some of you may even have earned a degree in another field. Many R.N. candidates already have some working experience in the health care field. Regardless of their academic and professional background, most nursing students find nursing exams to be very different from other exams they have taken—and very difficult. Why are nursing exams so hard?

> # Nursing exams are difficult because the questions ask you to make judgments and apply information—not just recall facts.

No matter how hard you study or how much information you can recall, you will not pass unless you can apply your nursing knowledge and make good nursing judgments on the exam.

Another reason nursing exams seem difficult is because the questions are written at what nurse educators refer to as a "high cognitive level." In other words, the questions seem difficult because they are designed to be difficult to answer! The complex questions on nursing exams are designed to test problem-solving and critical-thinking skills, as well as mastery of the nursing content. To prepare you to become a professional nurse, these exams must assess your ability to **identify problems in clinical situations, apply nursing principles, set nursing priorities, and evaluate nursing care.** The questions are complex because such decisions are **rarely black and white.**

WHY DO I SUDDENLY NEED NEW TEST-TAKING SKILLS?

Multiple-choice testing is here to stay, in nursing courses and in professional certification at all levels. The NCLEX-RN has developed its own distinctive characteristics because the nursing profession is so specialized. Many nursing course exams now use questions similar to those on the NCLEX-RN and other professional examinations to better prepare students for the NCLEX-RN. Every nursing student, therefore, needs specialized test-taking skills **to correctly interpret and answer the unique kinds of questions found on nursing exams.**

Have you had trouble selecting the correct answer to questions that present a clinical scenario and ask you to "identify the manifestation to which the nurse would give immediate attention?" Or have you found it confusing when asked to "select the highest (or lowest) priority nursing intervention" in a certain clinical scenario? Such questions are asking you to solve a problem. In nursing, problem-solving entails figuring out what the nurse should (or shouldn't) do when providing care to a client. Many nursing students find it hard to understand these questions.

Sometimes a question may present so much information about a clinical situation that it is difficult to determine which factors are most important. Or a question may seem to have two, three, or even four correct answers. Although students often regard these as "trick" questions, they are actually using a special kind of test-taking logic.

> **In a clinical situation, many actions might be appropriate. On an exam only one will be the best or priority action. This is how the exam tests your nursing judgment, as well as your nursing knowledge. It is very important to know how to go about answering judgment questions!**

You also need new skills because you need to be prepared to answer the many **different questions** that relate to a given clinical area. For example, there may be communication questions in addition to questions about pathophysiology, pharmacology, and nursing interventions and their rationales. These questions are included because therapeutic communication is so important in the safe and effective practice of nursing. An exam designed to test your knowledge in a specific clinical area will, therefore, be likely to include communication questions involving that area. Sometimes NCLEX-RN candidates report finding a great many psych questions on the NCLEX-RN, many of which were really communication questions. There are similar questions that test your ability to do client teaching. You need to be able to identify these questions and know what they are really about!

Other questions test your nursing knowledge about safety or infection control, or providing care to infants and children, pregnant clients and new mothers, elderly clients, clients with sensory impairments, confused clients, or other clients with special needs. On nursing exams, you may be called upon to apply your knowledge of everything from body mechanics to growth and development to special diets. This is especially true on the NCLEX-RN.

For these reasons, you need to know how to prepare for such comprehensive exams. You need to know how to answer all these special types of questions. In addition to reviewing nursing content, your preparation for either a course exam or the NCLEX-RN should include a plan for improving your test-taking skills and practice in answering problem-solving questions. *Test Question Logic (TQLogic™) for the NCLEX-RN Exam* will show you how to plan your review and how to answer the difficult questions you will find on your exams.

WILL THIS BOOK HELP ME BECOME A BETTER NURSE?

Yes! Questions on nursing exams are written at a high cognitive level because they use the nursing process. *Test Question Logic (TQLogic™) for the NCLEX-RN Exam* is designed specifically for nursing students. It continually emphasizes the nursing process because this is how nurses apply their nursing knowledge and make clinical decisions.

As you will see in Chapter Two, "Your Personalized Study Program for Nursing Exams," your comprehensive review for a nursing exam or the NCLEX-RN will need to include, among other things, early and late manifestations, pathophysiology, pharmacology, treatments, side and adverse effects, complications, client teaching, diet, comfort and safety measures, infection control, and other specific nursing measures. In the vocabulary of the nursing process, you will need to know how to assess a client and analyze data, how to plan nursing care, and how to implement and evaluate that care. You also need to know how to prioritize, how to assess safety risks, and how to communicate therapeutically. You need to know these things not just to answer test questions, but to be an effective nurse.

Nursing educators believe that testing is an essential component of the learning process. The nurse educators at MEDS are convinced that improved methods of reviewing nursing content and learning problem-solving skills enhance critical thinking ability where it counts most—on exams and in clinical situations.

WHAT WILL I GET OUT OF THIS BOOK?

The good news is that becoming a test-wise nursing student or NCLEX-RN Exam candidate is a skill you can learn! *Test Question Logic (TQLogic™) for the NCLEX-RN Exam* is the only nursing test-taking manual that teaches a unique method for correctly interpreting test questions. MEDS' Test Question Logic (TQLogic™) is a learning methodology for how to approach a test question. It helps students read and interpret test questions correctly, eliminate distractors, and use critical thinking. It breaks down answering test questions into three easy steps. First, identify the critical elements of a question such as:
· Key Words
· Who is the client?
· What is the issue/problem?
· What is the stem of the question asking?

All questions have four options of which three are distractors. It's often easy to eliminate two distractors; however, the remaining options typically appear equally correct. MEDS' TQLogic™ gives you strategies to deal with this scenario. The second step is to apply test-taking strategies such as:
· Identify a global response.
· Look for options with similar distractors.
· Look for options with similar words.

The third step is to apply nursing guidelines:
· Maslow's Hierarchy of Needs
· Nursing Process
· Communication Theory
· Teaching Learning Theory

If you apply the three steps of TQLogic™, you are on the path to NCLEX exam success. This method has enabled thousands of nursing students throughout the United States and Canada to increase their exam scores and to pass the NCLEX-RN on their first try.

Because this book is designed to help you master nursing exams and, most importantly, the NCLEX-RN Exam, the test-taking techniques presented in *Test*

Question Logic (TQLogic™) for the NCLEX-RN Exam use the nursing process. These techniques are designed to enhance and polish your professional problem-solving and critical-thinking skills. In addition, the study and review techniques presented should yield a time management payoff, a critical issue for so many of today's nursing students.

If you are an NCLEX-RN candidate, you need to become familiar with the unique NCLEX-RN format. You also need to practice using the strategies required to answer nursing questions. Chapter Nine, "How to Prepare for the NCLEX-RN Exam," will give you the **"inside scoop"** on the NCLEX-RN, answering all your questions about the exam and addressing your concerns. **"How can I review all the clinical areas, and how long will it take?" "Will I run out of time on the NCLEX-RN?" "How do I keep from 'reading into' a question?" "What kind of an answer is this question looking for?" "How can I choose between the two best options when both appear correct?" "What should I do when I'm just not sure of the answer?"** This book explains it all!

Be sure to note the special features of this book that are provided for maximum learning. **The drills in each chapter and the "Final Exam" in Chapter Ten let you practice your new test-taking skills and assess your progress. Chapter Eleven provides complete rationales for all the correct and incorrect options on the "Final Exam."**

Finally, the **CD-ROM** provided with this book offers you the opportunity to become familiar with the screen design and special format of the computerized NCLEX-RN Exam. We strongly recommend that you take advantage of this special option!

We invite you to view this presentation as a coaching session by an expert nurse educator who will offer you suggestions and guidelines. Nursing students and nurse educators, as well as NCLEX-RN candidates, will find this new and fresh approach extremely helpful. Here, finally, is an easy-to-follow book showing you how to **make the most of your nursing knowledge** on nursing exams. We are confident this book will give you the skills you need to improve your test scores and "ace" the NCLEX-RN. We hope you will enjoy *Test Question Logic (TQLogic™) for the NCLEX-RN Exam.*

Patricia A. Hoefler, M.S.N., R.N.
Program Director
MEDS Publishing

Chapter 1

HOW TO USE THIS BOOK

Test Question Logic (TQLogic™) for the NCLEX-RN Exam is specifically designed to teach you the specialized skills you need to maximize your scores on nursing course exams and the NCLEX-RN Exam.

This book will show you how to apply TQLogic:

✓ Use a proven method to correctly interpret multiple-choice nursing test questions.

✓ Use test-taking strategies to eliminate distractors and select the correct answer.

✓ Apply specific guidelines to answer the special kinds of questions you are certain to find on your exams: communication questions, questions that select priorities, and questions that use the nursing process.

✓ Learn and practice problem-solving skills.

✓ Plan your review of the nursing content to be covered on the NCLEX-RN or your nursing course exam.

✓ Pace yourself on a timed exam.

✓ Answer questions using the computerized NCLEX-RN format.

> **Whether you are a nursing student preparing for a course exam or a nursing graduate preparing for the NCLEX-RN Exam, we recommend that you take a few moments to familiarize yourself with the format of this book.**

First, if you have not yet done so, go back and read the **introduction,** "Why a Book on Problem-Solving and Test-Taking for Nursing Exams?" The introduction includes some useful information about the different kinds of questions used on nursing exams and will help you to understand what *Test Question Logic (TQLogic™) for the NCLEX-RN Exam* is designed to do for you. Then, look over the **table of contents** for an overview of the book's overall plan.

Nursing students should read **Chapter Two,** "Your Personalized Study Program for Nursing Exams." This will show you how to review material and prepare for a nursing exam. If you are a nursing graduate, turn instead to **Chapter Nine,** "How to Prepare for the NCLEX-RN." These two chapters will explain how to plan your review and how to use practice test questions. You may wish to read **Chapter Two** or **Chapter Nine** quickly now, to provide a context for learning the test-taking techniques and strategies in **Chapters Three** through **Seven,** and then return and read them in greater detail when you are actually planning your review. For now, be sure to note that the study methods outlined for both the NCLEX-RN and nursing course exams incorporate the nursing process.

Next, read **Chapters Three** through **Seven** carefully, in detail, and in the order that they occur in the book. These are the chapters on test-taking strategies. The first is **Chapter Three,** "How Do I Avoid 'Reading Into' a Test Question?" Students "read into" a test question because they are not able to interpret it correctly. This chapter explains how a test question is constructed and explains the unique "test-question logic" used in nursing exams. This chapter is the most basic and the most important of the chapters on test-taking strategies.

Chapter Four, "How Do I Choose Between the Two Best Options?" shows you how to use three powerful strategies for choosing the best option when two or more options appear equally correct, or when you aren't sure of the answer using your nursing knowledge alone. There is only one best option in each question. These strategies will help you to identify it.

Haven't you sometimes wondered what is being tested in communication questions? There are several pitfalls you can learn to avoid. **Chapter Five,** "Learning to Answer Communication Questions," provides useful insights into what makes these questions tick and gives you some simple guidelines to follow when selecting your answer.

"What is the priority nursing action at this time?" The answer depends on the clinical scenario, on what the question is asking, and on the options given. **Chapter Six,** "Learning to Answer Questions that Select Priorities," will show you how to apply four different priority-setting guidelines to test questions, including Maslow's hierarchy of needs. This chapter is ESSENTIAL for your success on the NCLEX-RN. If you are a nursing student, learn these guidelines now and use them on your course exams. Priority-setting questions don't have to be confusing.

Chapter Seven, "Learning to Answer Questions that Use the Nursing Process," focuses on the nursing process as a problem-solving and test-taking guideline and on key words that are signals to apply the nursing process when selecting the answer to a test question. This chapter is vital for NCLEX-RN candidates and also can save students a lot of trouble on their nursing course exams.

When taking a timed exam, it is important to pace yourself so that you will have time to complete the exam without undue stress and without getting marooned on any one question. In **Chapter Eight,** "How to Take a Timed Nursing Exam," you will learn how to use a simple pacing method and how to use sets of practice questions to increase your test-taking speed. NCLEX-RN candidates also will benefit from this chapter because there is a time limit on the NCLEX-RN and because good pacing reduces stress and improves concentration. Using a pacing technique when answering practice questions helps build speed, polish test-taking technique, and increases confidence.

Preparing for the NCLEX-RN can be overwhelming! **Chapter Nine,** "How to Prepare for the NCLEX-RN," gives you a simple outline to follow in designing your review. It explains the best way to study and how to use practice questions in your review.

> **When you have completed the chapters on test-taking strategies, be sure to take the Final Exams in Chapter 10 and 11. The *Test Smart* CD-ROM offers the same exams in a computerized format with bonus test-taking tips and instant scoring!**

Try the computerized format on your home computer or in your school's learning lab. It includes a Personal Performance Analysis, which shows how well you are doing at interpreting test questions, using test-taking strategies, applying prioritizing guidelines, using the nursing process, answering communication questions, and demonstrating your knowledge in each of the clinical areas.

For maximum learning, **Chapter Eleven,** "Answers and Analyses," provides complete rationales for each correct and incorrect answer to every question in the Final Exam. These complete rationales are hallmarks of MEDS. Test-taking tips are also provided. In the post-test segment of the disk, the program "remembers" which option you chose for each question and then lets you view rationales for each correct and incorrect option. The written exam format also includes complete rationales; they are provided in **Chapter Eleven.**

Chapter Twelve provides a summary of test-taking tips and strategies for preparing for the NCLEX-RN Exam. Everything from study tips to the NCLEX Exam Test Plan can be found here.

Chapter Thirteen gives an overview of Alternate Test Item Formats. The different formats are described, and an example is shown of each.

This brief guided tour of *Test Question Logic (TQLogic™) for the NCLEX-RN Exam* should give you a good idea of what you will learn and how you can use it. To begin, turn to **Chapter Two** (for nursing students) or **Chapter Nine** (for NCLEX-RN candidates). Whether you are using this book in a nursing class or on your own, you are already well on your way to improving your scores on nursing exams and passing the NCLEX-RN on your first try!

Chapter 2

YOUR PERSONALIZED STUDY PROGRAM FOR NURSING EXAMS

Isn't it true that you begin your preparation for a nursing exam on the first day of class? After all, don't you usually review your class notes when you review for an exam? You are anticipating an exam when you take notes and ask questions in class, and when you read assigned chapters in your textbook. By planning to use good preparation, note-taking, and review techniques, you can save time and be more successful.

Time Management: *Preparing for Class*

Students today are very busy, and many complain that they never have time to read the text ahead of time. It is very important, however, to prepare for class. Even if you have only a few minutes to spend, a little preparation will go a long way to increase your understanding of the material.

> **Preparation will pay off in terms of better comprehension and time you will save later. In fact, studies have shown that it can cut your study time in half. So be sure to prepare!**

First, **skim the chapter and read the subheadings** to get an overview of what is being covered. Then, **look at any charts or illustrations and read the captions.** Certainly you can plan to do at least this much before class!

Allow yourself the time to read the chapter through once, quickly. Look for basic concepts and the most important information. Make note of any questions you may have. Your goal as you prepare for class is **understanding the material, not memorizing it.**

Reading quickly and trying to get a good overview of the material will save you time now, and it will improve your memory and your comprehension. This important principle is the foundation of expensive "speed-reading" courses you may have seen advertised. Try it—it works!

When you have finished your first reading, look again at the subheadings and illustrations. This will reinforce the structure of the material presented and refresh your memory of the information you have covered.

How to Take Notes in Class

Your nursing instructor, in presenting material, is trying to make the material easier to understand. The instructor will, therefore, include explanations and clarifications of concepts and information covered in your textbook. When taking notes, your object should also be to **clarify.** Here are some basic principles:

Always be sure you know what is being discussed. This may seem obvious, but it isn't always simple to describe the subject of a discussion. Here are some possible topics related to the study of a health problem:

- Incidence

- Pathophysiological process

- Manifestations

- Side effects and adverse effects of treatments

- Complications

- Nursing interventions, including prioritizing

- Client teaching

Be sure you understand the rationale for a treatment or intervention. Your objective here is understanding. Although you can return to the textbook later for the details, **be sure to ask a question if there is something you don't understand.** Keep in mind that if something is not clear to you, it is probably unclear to others as well—especially if you have prepared for the class. Asking questions in class can decrease your study time by half!

Make sure you understand the priorities. What is most important? One clue would be any visual aids the instructor uses, such as charts, illustrations, or notes written on the board.

Be alert for the answers to any questions you may have had while reading the assigned material. If you have a question that is not answered during the course of the instructor's presentation, take the opportunity to ask it. Never leave a classroom if you are unclear about the information!

When you are taking notes, stay focused on the topic and try to be analytical. Note taking is not the same as taking dictation! **You should not be trying to write down everything the instructor says. If you have difficulty following the instructor, try bringing a tape recorder instead of trying to write everything down.**

After class, preferably the same day or the next, quickly review your class notes and the assigned textbook material and re-read any difficult sections of the text. Write down any remaining questions you have, and be sure to ask the instructor at the next class.

Reviewing for the Exam

Now it's exam time! You have your class notes and your textbook. How are you going to study for the exam?

Don't wait until the last minute! Take a calendar and plan the content you need to review, how long it will take, and exactly when you will do it. All Fortune 500 executives use personalized written plans for important projects. Putting your plan in writing is like writing your own personal guarantee of success! So write out your plan. If possible, plan to do your reviewing in the library or anywhere else you can be sure not to be interrupted.

Here is a comprehensive, time-saving way to review:

Review your class notes, paying special attention to rationales for interventions. If any are unclear, look them up in your text. As you review the material, keep in mind the phases of the **nursing process:** What should the nurse **assess**? How should the nurse **analyze** the assessment data? How should the nurse **plan** care for the client? What should the nurse keep in mind when **implementing** care? How should the nurse monitor and **evaluate** the client's response to therapy? Again, your focus is on **understanding,** so try to use your own words.

Look through the textbook. You may wish to make a brief, one-page outline of the subject, noting any areas that are particularly difficult for you. Are you familiar with the main points? Do you understand the charts and illustrations? Reread any sections that you found unclear. If you complete your preparation ahead of time and have questions about the material, **ask your instructor!**

Use some of the review aids that are available in your bookstore or learning lab. For example, look for audio tapes and video tapes for review of all clinical areas, plus special topics such as pharmacology and safety. These tapes are especially useful when reviewing for final exams, when a great deal of material is to be covered at one time.

Use practice questions. This is extremely important! **Practice questions assess and reinforce what you have learned.** Practice questions reflect what goes on in real clinical situations, and they help you to become more analytical.

Teamwork harnesses brainpower—if you can, **study in teams with other good students.** Group study is good for morale, too!

Using Practice Questions

Be sure to plan time during your review to **answer practice questions** covering the subject.

> **Answering practice questions is as important as going over your notes or reviewing your text because it gives you a chance to practice applying your newly acquired nursing knowledge.**

As a rule of thumb, plan to answer about 200 practice questions in preparation for a typical 50-question exam. You will find "Q&A" (question and answer) books in your bookstore, as well as in your learning lab or library. Computerized practice tests are also available. When answering questions, be sure to time yourself and practice **pacing** yourself (see Chapter Eight, "How to Take a Timed Nursing Exam").

To assess your knowledge and your test-taking skills, be sure to check your answers and read the rationales! Assess the reason why you answered any questions incorrectly. Did you misunderstand or "read into" the question? Did you lack the required nursing knowledge to answer the question? Is there a test-taking strategy that would have helped you to select the correct answer?

Finally, when you have completed a set of practice questions, you may wish to return to your textbook or class notes and review any information that gave you difficulty. You may also wish to return to *Successful Problem-Solving and Test-Taking* to review how to answer particular types of questions or how to use certain test-taking strategies.

The Payoff!

Following these guidelines for organized, streamlined preparation and review will pay off in increased confidence, increased understanding, better use of your time, and increased test scores. Try it and see!

NOTES

Chapter 3

HOW DO I AVOID "READING INTO" THE QUESTION?

It seems justified to lose points on an exam because you did not know the necessary information. It is extremely frustrating, however, to score poorly on an exam because you "read into" or misread the questions!

You can maximize your score on your nursing course exams and the NCLEX-RN Exam by learning some test-taking techniques and strategies. This chapter will show you some techniques to help you to read and interpret test questions correctly and help you eliminate incorrect options.

A three-step technique is described in this chapter:

FIRST, you will learn a technique for analyzing a test question by separating what the **case scenario** in the question **tells** you from what the **stem** of the question **asks**.

SECOND, you will learn a technique for interpreting a test question by identifying the **four critical elements**.

THIRD, you will learn a technique for **eliminating incorrect options**. Each time you answer a test question, you should use **all three** of these techniques.

IDENTIFYING THE "CASE SCENARIO" AND THE "STEM"

The first step in analyzing a test question is to separate what the question **tells** you from what it is **asking**.

Each test question basically consists of three parts:

1. A case scenario, which describes a clinical situation.

2. A stem, which asks you to select an answer.

3. Four options from which you must select the correct answer.

Here is a sample test question set up like a computerized NCLEX-RN screen showing the **case scenario,** the **stem** and the **four options.**

As you can see, this question **tells** you about a safety issue facing the nurse. The **case scenario** in the question **gives you the clinical information** you should consider when selecting the correct answer.

In preparing to administer a medication to a confused elderly client, the nurse discovers that the client does not have an identification bracelet on. The client states that the medication has already been taken. Which of the following nursing actions provides for the client's safety?

☐ 1. Ask if the client might be confused about taking the medication.

Case Scenario and Stem

☐ 2. Identify the client based upon which bed is occupied in the room.

☐ 3. Check the client's chart and ask another health care worker to identify the client.

☐ 4. Ask the client's name and then obtain an identification bracelet for the client.

Four Options

The **stem** is the portion of the test question that **asks** the nurse to solve a specific problem by selecting one of the **four options.** The **stem** in the question **asks** you to choose the option that presents the best action for safely administering medication to a confused client.

The **stem** usually comes **after** the **case scenario** and asks you a question referring to the case scenario statement. Here is another sample test question with the stem in bold print:

> A client had a cerebral vascular accident two weeks ago and is paralyzed on the left side. While getting the client out of bed to sit in a wheelchair, **which nursing action is essential?**

Note that the case scenario and the stem are not always in separate sentences! Sometimes the case scenario seems to run into or overlap the stem, as it does in the above question. When this happens, you can still separate what the question is **telling** you from what it is specifically **asking**. It may be helpful in a question like this to restate the question in your own words. Here is the question restated and, again, the **stem** is in bold print:

> A client had a cerebral vascular accident two weeks ago and is paralyzed on the left side. The nurse must get the client out of bed and into a wheelchair. **Which nursing action is essential in making such a transfer?**

Now here is another question about the same client, with the **case scenario** in bold print:

> **A client had a cerebral vascular accident two weeks ago and is paralyzed on the left side. In transferring the client to a wheelchair, the nurse notices a reddened area on the left hip.** Which nursing action is essential?

Notice that, although the stem still asks you to select an essential nursing action, the **case scenario** has been changed. It is very important to **read all the information in the case scenario!** The second question about the client will have a different answer from the first question.

It is important to identify what the question *tells* you and what it *asks* because:

1. Incorrect options may "answer" something that is not actually being asked.

2. Incorrect options may assume information that was not given in the case scenario.

3. Reading each question carefully will help you make the most of your nursing knowledge.

Some questions may not describe a specific clinical situation. For example, a question without a case scenario statement might simply ask you to select the option that best:

- Identifies a manifestation of a specific disease

- Describes the difference between two diseases

- Identifies a problem

- Specifies the priority nursing action for a certain situation

You can think of a question **without a case scenario** statement as giving you a **subject with the stem.** The stem of such a question asks you something regarding that subject.

Here is a sample test question set up like the computerized NCLEX-RN screen showing the **subject with stem** and the **four options.**

Remotivation therapy is used in long-term care facilities for which of the following reasons?   ↖ *Subject with Stem*

☐ 1. Stimulate and encourage social participation.

☐ 2. Reorient clients with cognitive problems.

☐ 3. Share memories of past experiences and events.

☐ 4. Resolve emotional problems.   ↖ *Four Options*

IDENTIFYING THE FOUR CRITICAL ELEMENTS

Learning to identify the critical elements in a test question is crucial to interpreting the question correctly.

> ## The four critical elements in each test question are the:
>
> 1. Key words
> 2. Client
> 3. Issue
> 4. Type of stem

1. What are the *key words?*

Key words are the important words or phrases in a question. Key words focus your attention on crucial ideas in the stem and in the options. Here are some phrases from questions with the key words in **bold** print:

> - **Early** or **late** manifestations
> - **Immediately** after surgery or in the **postoperative** period
> - The **most likely** or **least likely** characteristics to occur
> - The **initial** nursing action
> - **After several days**
> - **On the day of** admission

It's important to be able to recognize **key words** because a common type of distractor is a statement that would be correct if the **key words** were missing or different. For instance, a question that asks you to select **early** manifestations of a complication may contain as a distractor an option that lists several **late** manifestations of the complication.

2. Who is the *client* in the question?

The client is the person who is the focus of the question. The following are examples of who the client may be:

- The person with the health problem

- The person specifically identified in the question as the "client"

- A relative or friend of the person with the health problem

- Another client in the health care setting

- Another staff nurse

- A nursing assistant

It is crucial to identify the client in the question because the answer must relate to the client.

3. What is the *issue* in the question?

The **issue** is the specific problem or subject about which the question is <u>asking</u>. For example, the issue might be a:

- Drug (e.g., digoxin, [Lanoxin])
- Problem (e.g., drug addiction, depression)
- Toxic effect of a drug (e.g., nausea, vomiting)
- Behavior (e.g., restlessness, agitation)
- Disorder (e.g., diabetes mellitus, ulcerative colitis)
- Procedure (e.g., glucose tolerance test, cardiac catheterization)

4. What is the *type of stem?*

As we have explained, the stem is the part of the question that asks you to solve a problem and select a response. To select the correct option, you need to determine the **type of stem.**

There are two types of stems:

A.   TRUE RESPONSE STEMS

B.   FALSE RESPONSE STEMS

True response stems are questions for which the answer would be an **appropriate** nursing action or an **accurate** explanation. For example, **a true response stem might ask you to identify:**

- An **appropriate** nursing action
- The **most essential or highest priority** nursing action
- A **safe** nursing judgment
- A **therapeutic** nursing response
- An **accurate** rationale for a nursing action
- An action or statement by the client **indicating the success** of the nurse's client teaching
- A **correct explanation** of the difference between two disorders

In the examples shown below, note the words in **bold** print. These words focus your attention on the "best" or "most correct" option. **Here are some examples of true response stems:**

- Which interpretation of these findings by the nurse is **most** justifiable?
- Which nursing action is **most** important?
- The nurse would demonstrate the **best** judgment by taking which action?
- During the early period, which nursing intervention would be **best**?
- **Initially,** the nurse **should:**
- The nurse understands that the **chief** purpose of the drug is to:
- The nurse should give **immediate** consideration to which manifestation?
- The nurse understands that the client is **at risk** for which complication?
- In caring for an adolescent male client, the nurse understands that, as compared to preadolescent boys, **most** adolescent boys **need:**
- Which finding would the nurse identify as **consistent** with the admitting diagnosis?
- The nurse knows that the **similar** characteristic for the client with infectious hepatitis and the client in the first trimester of pregnancy is:
- The nurse **knows that the client understands** how to care for the health problem when the client:

False response stems are those for which the answer would generally be an **inappropriate** nursing action or an **inaccurate** explanation. For example, **a false response stem might ask you to identify:**

- An action the nurse **should avoid.**
- The **least essential** or **lowest priority** nursing action.
- A nursing action that **fails to address** the client's problem.
- An **unsafe** nursing judgment.
- A **nontherapeutic** nursing response.
- An **inadequate** or incorrect rationale for a nursing action.
- An **inaccurate** explanation of the difference between two disorders.
- A statement or action by which the client indicates a **lack of motivation or understanding** of how to care for a health problem.

In other words, a **false response stem** asks you to select an answer that is **wrong** or that **has something negative or unimportant about it.**

The following are examples of false response stems. Note the negative word or phrase in **bold** print:

> • At this time, which nursing action would **place the client at risk**?
>
> • The nurse knows that which medication would be **contraindicated** for this client?
>
> • The nurse should advise the client to **avoid** taking the medication with:
>
> • The **least important** concern for the nurse to raise with the client at this time is:
>
> • Which nursing action receives the **lowest priority** at this time?
>
> • The nurse would identify that the client **requires further instruction** in CPR if the client's hands are placed:
>
> • Which nursing action would demonstrate an **unsafe** nursing judgement?
>
> • The nurse knows that which manifestation is an unexpected finding associated with hypertension?

ELIMINATING INCORRECT OPTIONS

After you have identified the four critical elements in a test question, then you can begin to narrow your choices for selecting the correct option. All questions on the NCLEX-RN Exam, and most multiple choice questions that you will find on your nursing course exams, have four options. Of these, three are "distractors" and one is the correct answer.

> **"Distractors" are incorrect options that are designed to resemble the correct answer. They are intended to "distract" you from answering correctly.**

Here is a selection procedure to help you eliminate the distractors.

1. First, decide whether the question has a **true response stem** or a **false response stem.**

2. Then, read each of the four options to determine whether it is appropriate/ correct or inappropriate/incorrect (i.e., whether it is a true statement or not).

For a *true response stem,* make a decision about each option as follows:

+ This might be the **correct answer** because this option is **appropriate.**

– This is a **distractor** because this option is **inappropriate.**

? This is a **possibility** because I am **not sure.**

For a *false response stem,* make a decision about each option as follows:

+ This might be the **correct answer** because this option is **inappropriate.**

– This is a **distractor** because this option is **appropriate.**

? This is a **possibility** because I am **not sure.**

Sometimes, just applying the test-taking techniques described in this chapter and narrowing your choices for selecting the correct option in the manner described above leads directly to the correct option! When it doesn't, some strategies you will learn in Chapter Four can help you narrow the choices even further.

HOW TO AVOID MISREADING TEST QUESTIONS

Misreading test questions is a major problem that hinders success on nursing exams. There are many ways in which a question can be misread!

Misreading a test question may happen because you:

1. Incorrectly analyze what the question is really asking

2. Overlook key words such as "early," "late," "unsafe," or "inappropriate"

3. "Read into" a question information that is not actually given

4. Incorrectly interpret a disorder (for example, mistakenly interpreting a complication of diabetes mellitus, such as ketoacidosis, as diabetes mellitus itself)

Here are some tips to help you avoid misreading test questions:

1. Avoid incorrectly analyzing what is being asked:
   - Separate the case scenario and the stem
   - Identify the client
   - Identify the issue
   - Identify the type of stem
2. Avoid overlooking important words: **identify the key words.**
3. Avoid "reading into" a question:
   Try to restate the question in your own words. Then eliminate any option that includes "new" information about the client or the clinical situation that was not given in the case scenario. You should also eliminate any option that requires you to make assumptions about the client involving information not presented in the case scenario.
4. Avoid misinterpreting disorders:
   Review carefully for the exam! Use the method outlined in Chapter Two to review for nursing course exams. For the NCLEX-RN Exam, be sure to follow the plan in Chapter Nine. Focus on any areas in which you have difficulty. Then, use your nursing knowledge and your test-taking techniques when you read each question.

Guidelines to Use When Narrowing the Options

- Make a decision about each option as you read it—you will save time.
- You should be able to eliminate at least two options by using this selection procedure.
- After you have eliminated an option, do not go back to it. Continue to work with the remaining options.
- If you are left with one ➕ option and one ❓ option, select the ➕ as the correct answer. Remember to always go with what you know!
- Using a selection procedure allows you to make an educated guess when necessary. If you are left with two, you have a 50% chance of guessing correctly. If you make a wild guess from all four choices, you have only a 25% chance of guessing correctly.

Practice Session: Identifying the Critical Elements and Eliminating Options

As you answer the following questions, remember to ask yourself these questions:

1. What are the key words?

2. Who is the client?

3. What is the issue?

4. What is the stem asking?

Always be sure to determine whether the question has a true response stem or a false response stem. When you know the type of stem, then make a decision about each of the options as you read them by using the selection procedure. After you have answered the question, read the analysis. Note that the **key words** and the **correct answer** are in bold print.

DRILL 1

The nurse is admitting a client suspected of having diabetes mellitus. The nurse would expect to observe:

1. Shallow, labored respirations.
2. Increased blood pressure associated with slight periorbital edema.
3. Periods of altered pulse rate.
4. Increased urinary output.

ANALYSIS 1

Critical Elements	
Key words:	See bold print
Client:	A client with diabetes mellitus
Issue:	A characteristic of diabetes mellitus
Type of Stem:	True response stem

Eliminate Options

The nurse is admitting a client suspected of having **diabetes mellitus.** The nurse would **expect** to **observe:**

1. Shallow, labored respirations.
   Were you tempted by this option? This is a good distractor! It might appear to be a possibility if you thought this was Kussmaul's breathing. However, Kussmaul's breathing is a characteristic of ketoacidosis, which is a complication of diabetes mellitus. This question is about a characteristic of diabetes, not a complication of diabetes. In addition, Kussmaul's breathing is deep and rapid, not shallow and labored.

2. Increased blood pressure associated with slight periorbital edema.
   This is NOT *a characteristic of diabetes.*

3. Periods of altered pulse rate.
   This is a sign of ketoacidosis—a complication of diabetes—so you may have thought this was another possibility. This is another DISTRACTOR, however, because the question specifically asks for a characteristic of diabetes.

4. **Increased urinary output.**
   This option is correct. It is THE ONLY CHARACTERISTIC OF DIABETES *presented in these four options. Remember the three Ps associated with the diagnosis of diabetes mellitus, which are polyuria, polyphagia and polydypsia.*

In assessing an adult client with diabetes mellitus, the nurse would identify which finding to be inconsistent with this diagnosis?

2 DRILL

1. Increased body weight.
2. Increased urinary output.
3. Periods of polydypsia.
4. Alterations in heart rate and rhythm.

2 ANALYSIS

Critical Elements	
Key words:	See bold print
Client:	An adult client
Issue:	A finding that would NOT be observed in an adult with diabetes mellitus
Type of Stem:	False response stem

Eliminate Options

In assessing an **adult** client with **diabetes mellitus**, the nurse would identify which finding to be **inconsistent** with this diagnosis?

□ 1. Increased body weight.
Since the adult diabetic gains weight, this finding would be EXPECTED with the diagnosis. The false response stem in this question asks for a finding that would be UNEXPECTED. This option is a distractor.

□ 2. Increased urinary output.
Since we are looking for an UNEXPECTED finding, this a distractor and not the answer. This is an EXPECTED manifestation of adult diabetes.

□ 3. Periods of polydypsia.
This is an EXPECTED manifestation of adult diabetes. Since we are looking for an UNEXPECTED finding, this is not the answer.

⊞ **4. Alterations heart rate and rhythm.**
This question has a false response stem, so the answer is something that the nurse would NOT expect to find in an adult diabetic. Altered heart rate and rhythm are NOT characteristic of diabetes. The other three options are distractors: they list manifestations consistent with the diagnosis of adult diabetes mellitus.

DRILL 3

The nurse caring for a client with urolithiasis knows which nursing intervention would be inappropriate?

1. Forcing fluids.
2. Straining the urine.
3. Complete bed rest.
4. Medication for colic or discomfort.

ANALYSIS 3

Critical Elements	
Key words:	See bold print
Client:	A client with urolithiasis
Issue:	A nursing measure NOT included in the nursing care of a client with urolithiasis. (To help define urolithiasis, dissect the word: "uro-" is kidney and "lithiasis" is stone)
Type of Stem:	False response stem

Eliminate Options

The nurse caring for a client with **urolithiasis** knows which nursing measure would be **inappropriate?**

◼ 1. Forcing fluids.
Nursing care for urolithiasis INCLUDES encouraging fluid intake to help flush out the kidney stone. This is a distractor.

◼ 2. Straining the urine.
Nursing care for urolithiasis INCLUDES obtaining the stones for analysis, so straining is necessary.

✚ **3. Complete bed rest.**
This is the answer to this question with a FALSE RESPONSE stem. Complete bed rest is INAPPROPRIATE because the client may ambulate. Ambulation helps the stone to pass through the kidney.

◼ 4. Medication for colic or discomfort.
This is another DISTRACTOR because nursing care for urolithiasis INCLUDES medicating for pain, which can be severe. Remember, the answer is something that is incorrect in the care of a client with a kidney stone.

A client was admitted for a severe episode of gastrointestinal bleeding. Prior to discharge, which statement by the client would indicate to the nurse the need for further instruction?

4 DRILL

1. "If my arthritis bothers me, I can take acetaminophen (Tylenol)."
2. "I'm glad I gave up drinking five years ago."
3. "I can't wait to get home so I can have my morning coffee."
4. "I'll take my cimetidine (Tagamet) before eating and at bedtime."

4 ANALYSIS

Critical Elements	
Key words:	See bold print
Client:	A client with gastrointestinal bleeding
Issue:	A statement by the client that indicates a lack of understanding about self-care after an episode of gastrointestinal bleeding
Type of Stem:	False response stem

Eliminate Options

A client was admitted for a **severe** episode of **gastrointestinal bleeding.** Prior to discharge, which statement by the client would indicate to the nurse that the client **needs further instruction?**

▬ 1. "If my arthritis bothers me, I'll take acetaminophen (Tylenol)."
Using Tylenol is APPROPRIATE *for this client (although any aspirin-related drug would be contraindicated because it causes GI bleeding). The stem asks you to identify a statement that indicates that the client* DOES NOT UNDERSTAND *how to care for this health-care problem.*

▬ 2. "I'm glad I gave up drinking five years ago."
The client's statement indicates AN UNDERSTANDING *that caring for this health problem requires avoiding alcohol. Alcohol stimulates the GI tract. Look for a statement indicating that the client* DOES NOT UNDERSTAND *what to do.*

➕ 3. **"I can't wait to get home so I can have my morning coffee."**
This is the correct answer because such a statement by the client indicates a LACK OF UNDERSTANDING *of how to care for this health problem. Coffee stimulates the GI tract, and it* SHOULD BE AVOIDED. *This response shows that the client* NEEDS FURTHER EDUCATION. *This is the type of question that can be easily misread!*

◼ 4. "I'll take my cimetidine (Tagamet) before eating and at bedtime."
*The client CORRECTLY intends to take the Tagamet before eating
and at bedtime. Tagamet is used in the treatment of peptic ulcers to
inhibit the secretion of histamine.*

DRILL 5

The nurse understands that, physiologically, the difference between angina and myocardial infarction is that with angina:

1. Arterial perfusion is briefly inadequate. With a myocardial infarction,
    arterial perfusion is cut off permanently.
2. The enzymes SGOT, LDH, and CPK are elevated. After a myocardial
    infarction, they are not elevated.
3. Adrenocorticosteroids are released to reduce the inflammatory re-
    action. With a myocardial infarction, these hormones are absent.
4. Hypertension and congestive heart failure are absent. With a myo-
    cardial infarction, hypertension and congestive heart failure are
    present.

ANALYSIS 5

Critical Elements	
Key words:	See bold print
Client:	Any client with a myocardial infarction or angina
Issue:	The physiological difference between angina and myocardial infarction (Note: This is an example of a question that does not have a case scenario.)
Type of Stem:	True response stem

Eliminate Options

The nurse understands that, **physiologically**, the **difference** between
angina and myocardial infarction is:

➕ 1. **With angina, arterial perfusion is briefly inadequate. With a myo-
       cardial infarction, arterial perfusion is cut off permanently.**
       *This is an ACCURATE comparison, because in a myocardial infarc-
       tion the blockage of arterial perfusion is permanent and angina in-
       volves only temporarily inadequate arterial perfusion. Note: Even
       though this answer is accurate, you should always read all four
       options to make sure this one is the best.*

2. With angina, the enzymes SGOT, LDH, and CPK are elevated. After a myocardial infarction, they are not elevated.
This is an INACCURATE *comparison; actually, the opposite is true. With an infarction, the enzymes are elevated. Because there is no muscle or tissue damage in angina, the enzymes are not elevated. This is a distractor.*

3. With angina, adrenocorticosteroids are released to reduce the inflammatory reaction. With a myocardial infarction, these hormones are absent.
This is a good DISTRACTOR, *because it looks like it might be a possible answer. However, this comparison is inaccurate. There is no inflammatory reaction with a myocardial infarction. Did you know that? You probably did! When deciding between two options, always choose what you know for sure.*

4. With angina, hypertension and congestive heart failure are absent. With a myocardial infarction, hypertension and congestive heart failure are present.
Does this look like another POSSIBILITY *to you? These complications* MAY *be associated with either angina or a myocardial infarction, so this comparison is not valid.*

All four options in this question are lengthy, but this question is not too difficult. It may take some time to read, however, and you need to read each option carefully!

In contrast to the client with angina, the nurse will observe that the client with a myocardial infarction experiences:

1. Pain that is relieved by rest and nitroglycerin.
2. Possible signs of increased cardiac output and hypoxia.
3. Pain that occurs with increased stress and exercise.
4. Severe, crushing pain that begins spontaneously.

6 DRILL

Critical Elements

Key words:	See bold print
Client:	Any client with a myocardial infarction
Issue:	A manifestation of a myocardial infarction that is not found in angina
Type of Stem:	True response stem (comparison)

6 ANALYSIS

Eliminate Options

In **contrast** to the client with angina, the nurse will observe that the client with a **myocardial infarction** experiences:

1. Pain that is relieved by rest and nitroglycerin.
   This is a characteristic of angina that is NOT FOUND IN A MYOCARDIAL INFARCTION. *You are looking for just the opposite.*

2. Possible signs of increased cardiac output and hypoxia.
   This option may appear to be a POSSIBILITY. *It is true that hypoxia occurs with a myocardial infarction, and the word "possible" may tempt you to choose this option. But there are two manifestations in this option and, for the option to be correct, both must be associated with a myocardial infarction.* INCREASED CARDIAC OUTPUT *does not occur with a myocardial infarction; cardiac output is* DECREASED *due to the damaged muscle.*

3. Pain that occurs with increased stress and exercise.
   These are factors precipitating angina, they are NOT ASSOCIATED WITH MYOCARDIAL INFARCTION. *The question is asking for just the opposite.*

4. **Severe, crushing pain that begins spontaneously.**
   Although this type of pain does not occur with all myocardial infarctions, THIS IS MOST TYPICAL OF AN INFARCTION *and not angina. Anginal pain is usually provoked by stress or exercise. Pain associated with a myocardial infarction is usually severe and is not abated by the use of nitroglycerin.*

In caring for a client with ulcerative colitis, the nurse understands an important difference between a psychosomatic and a conversion disorder is that in the psychosomatic disorder the:

1. Physical manifestations are consciously selected by the person.
2. Physical manifestations are relieved when the mental conflict is resolved.
3. Physical manifestations may be fatal if left untreated.
4. Person characteristically has an attitude of indifference toward the physical manifestations.

Critical Elements

Key words:	See bold print
Client:	A client with ulcerative colitis
Issue:	An aspect of a psychosomatic disorder that does not apply to a conversion disorder.
Type of Stem:	True response stem (comparison)

Eliminate Options

In caring for a client with **ulcerative colitis,** the nurse understands an **important difference** between a psychosomatic and a **conversion** disorder is that **in the psychosomatic disorder the:**

■ 1. Physical manifestations are consciously selected by the person.
The physical manifestations are NOT CONSCIOUSLY SELECTED IN EITHER ILLNESS. *Look for an accurate statement about a psychosomatic disorder that is not true for a conversion disorder.*

？ 2. Physical manifestations are relieved when the mental conflict is resolved.
This a good distractor, because it might be a POSSIBILITY. *However, this is true of* BOTH *illnesses. In both psychosomatic and conversion disorders, the manifestations decrease as the mental conflict is relieved. The issue of the question is the* DIFFERENCE *between these two illnesses.*

✚ **3. Physical manifestations may be fatal if left untreated.**
This is the major difference between these two illnesses. The client with a psychophysiological (psychosomatic) disorder may die from the illness if there is no medical intervention. The client with a conversion disorder (a hypochondriac) will not die from the physical manifestations. Note that this question could have been asked without any reference to an actual client. The writer of this question tossed in a big clue by providing a client with ulcerative colitis, which can be life-threatening if it is not treated. That is another reason to identify key words: to take advantage of those free hints!

■ 4. The person characteristically has an attitude of indifference toward the physical manifestations.
This is NOT AN ACCURATE STATEMENT ABOUT A CLIENT WITH ULCERATIVE COLITIS, *who is most likely very concerned about their medical problem because it is life-threatening. This is a characteristic of a conversion disorder.*

In this chapter, three important strategies
were introduced. In addition to these strategies,
some important points when answering
test questions are listed below.

Points to Remember

- Answer questions **as if the situation were ideal,** and the nurse had **all the time and resources** needed. The only client you need to be concerned about is the one in the question!

- Be sure to identify the **false response stems,** that ask you to select an inappropriate nursing action or an inaccurate rationale or comparison. These questions are easy to **misread.**

- Lengthy questions are not always difficult! Read them carefully, and "go with what you know."

- Certain imprecise words, like ***"possible," "usually," or "may,"*** will often make a statement true and may make that option a "possible (?)" answer. On the other hand, absolute terms like *"always"* or *"never"* tend to make a statement incorrect.

- Always read all the options before selecting the best one!

- Make sure to read all of the options—and **then** select the best!

Chapter 4

HOW DO I CHOOSE BETWEEN THE TWO BEST OPTIONS?

In most nursing exam questions, often it is easy to eliminate two distractors. The two remaining options, however, often appear equally correct. For example, of four possible nursing interventions, two may be inappropriate and easily ruled out, but both of the remaining two may appear quite appropriate. Or you may have difficulty deciding between two possible options that appear to be very close in meaning. So how do you decide?

The following test-taking strategies will help you to choose between the two best options. If you are unable to choose the answer using your nursing knowledge, you should apply the strategies rather than just guess at the answer. In this chapter, **you will learn three strategies that will help you master the skill of eliminating incorrect options and choosing the correct answer.**

> **The test-taking strategies presented in this chapter will require that you understand the test-taking terminology and techniques presented in Chapter Three. If you have not yet read Chapter Three, do so before proceeding with Chapter Four.**

STRATEGY 1

THE GLOBAL RESPONSE

When more than one option appears to be correct, **look for a global response.**

> **A global response is one that is
> a general statement and may include
> the ideas of other options within it.**

This option is often the correct answer when two or three more specific options appear equally correct.

Practice Session: Looking for the Global Response

Read and answer the following questions, looking for an option that is more global than the others. First, review the questions by identifying the four critical elements. Then narrow your choices, and look for the option that includes a global response. After you have answered the question, read the analysis. Note that the **key words** and the **answer** are shown in **bold** print.

DRILL 1

The nurse understands that the overall aim of therapy for a client with cerebral palsy is to:

1. Improve muscle control and coordination.
2. Correct the underlying cause of the disease.
3. Prevent contractures and emotional disturbances.
4. Maximize the client's assets and minimize limitations.

ANALYSIS 1

Critical Elements	
Key words:	See bold print
Client:	Any client with cerebral palsy
Issue:	The overall aim of therapy for cerebral palsy
Type of Stem:	True response stem

Eliminate Options

The nurse understands that the **overall aim** of therapy for a client with **cerebral palsy** is to:

? 1. Improve muscle control and coordination.
This is an appropriate goal of therapy in cerebral palsy and a POSSI-BILITY. Since cerebral palsy causes spasticity of the muscles and gross and fine motor incoordination, muscle training is needed. By reading on, however, you can see that this is too specific and not global enough to be the best statement of the overall aim of therapy. Always make sure you read all the options before selecting the best one!

– 2. Correct the underlying cause of the disease.
This is an INAPPROPRIATE GOAL, *since cerebral palsy is a nonprogressive motor disorder that stems from permanent damage to the motor centers and pathways in the brain. Correcting the underlying cause is not medically possible.*

? 3. Prevent contractures and emotional disturbances.
This is a POSSIBILITY *and another good distractor, because it is an appropriate goal in cerebral palsy. This is one goal of therapy, since communication and self-help deficits and spasticity cause contractures and emotional problems. Like option 1, this is another specific goal.*

+ **4. Maximize the client's assets and minimize limitations.**
This is the best option because it is the most complete or global answer to the question. Note that this option encompasses the ideas of options 1 and 3.

2 DRILL

The nurse assigned to care for a child with cerebral palsy should obtain information concerning the child's abilities, limitations, interests and habits, because the aim of therapy is to:

1. Assess the child's assets and potentialities and capitalize on these in the rehabilitative process, while overlooking limitations.
2. Reverse abnormal functioning and restore brain function through rehabilitation.
3. Provide a therapeutic program that avoids subjecting the child to frustrating experiences that decrease achievement.
4. Develop an individualized therapeutic program that uses the child's assets and abilities to achieve success as well as develops the child's ability to cope with frustration and failure.

ANALYSIS

2

Critical Elements	
Key words:	See bold print
Client:	A child with cerebral palsy
Issue:	The aim of therapy for cerebral palsy
Type of Stem:	True response stem

Eliminate Options

The nurse who is assigned to care for a child with **cerebral palsy** should obtain information concerning the child's abilities, limitations, interests and habits because the **aim** of **therapy** is to:

■ 1. Assess the child's assets and potentialities and capitalize on these in the rehabilitative process while overlooking limitations.
   Part of the goal statement is appropriate, but part of it is INAPPROPRIATE, which makes the whole option incorrect. It is never an aim of therapy to overlook the client's limitations.

■ 2. Reverse abnormal functioning and restore brain function through rehabilitation.
   This is definitely an INAPPROPRIATE goal, since cerebral palsy results in permanent malfunction of the motor centers. Brain damage cannot be reversed or restored.

■ 3. Provide a therapeutic program that avoids subjecting the child to frustrating experiences that decrease achievement.
   This goal is INAPPROPRIATE because of the word "avoid." The aim of therapy is not to avoid a frustrating experience. This would be also be unrealistic.

✚ **4. Develop an individualized therapeutic program that uses the child's assets and abilities and provides experiences to achieve success as well as the ability to cope with frustration and failure.**
   This is an APPROPRIATE goal for cerebral palsy therapy. This is also a global option, since it includes recognizing the client's assets and helping the child to cope with frustrations and failures due to limitations. This is a lengthy option that is comprehensive.

A client says, "I am having a real problem getting pregnant. What could be wrong?" Which idea should be incorporated into the nurse's response?

1. Infertility is often caused by congenital anomalies of the reproductive organs.
2. Infertility is sometimes precipitated by the use of over-the-counter drugs.
3. Infertility is frequently caused by multiple factors rather than a single factor.
4. Emotional problems, including stress, can cause a decrease in fertility.

Critical Elements	
Key words:	See bold print
Client:	A client having difficulty conceiving
Issue:	Possible causes of infertility
Type of Stem:	True response stem

Eliminate Options

A client says, "I am having a **real problem getting pregnant.** What could be wrong?" Which ideas should be incorporated into the **nurse's response**?

1. Infertility is often caused by congenital anomalies of the reproductive organs.
   This is a POSSIBLE answer because the word "often" makes the information it contains true. However, this is just one possible factor, and the case scenario does not present much information about the client. Look for a more global response.

2. Infertility is sometimes precipitated by the use of over-the-counter drugs.
   This is another POSSIBLE answer because of the word "sometimes." Like option 1, however, this is just one possible cause.

3. **Infertility is frequently caused by multiple factors rather than a single factor.**
   This is the correct option because it is the most global. The "multiple factors" may include congenital anomalies, over-the-counter drugs, and emotional difficulties. When two options contain correct information but are very specific, with no reason to prefer one to the other, look for an option that is more global. This option is the most comprehensive.

4. Emotional difficulties, including stress, can cause a decrease in fertility. *This is another* POSSIBILITY *because the information it contains is correct. However, this option is also too specific.*

SIMILAR DISTRACTORS

If you don't know the answer, your second strategy is to look for similar distractors.

 Remember that there is only one best option.

If two options essentially say the same thing or include the same idea, then neither of these options can be the answer. The answer has to be the option that is different. Although this is a difficult strategy to understand, it is an excellent strategy to learn and use. The following questions will help to clarify this strategy.

Practice Session: Looking for Similar Distractors

Read and answer the following questions, eliminating the options that are similar. First, read the questions, identify the four critical elements and narrow your choices. Then, practice using the similar distractor strategy by looking for the option that is different. After you have answered the question, read the analysis. The **key words** and the **answer** are in **bold** print.

To monitor a client for the most common complication arising from the administration of total parenteral nutrition (TPN), the nurse should:

1. Weigh the client at the same time each day using the same scale.
2. Keep accurate records of total intake and total output.
3. Determine the increase or decrease in body weight each day.
4. Take the client's temperature at least every four hours.

Critical Elements

Key words: See bold print
Client: A client receiving total parenteral nutrition (TPN)
Issue: Monitoring for the most common complication from TPN
Type of Stem: True response stem

Eliminate Options

To **monitor** a client for the **most common complication** arising from the administration of **total parenteral nutrition (TPN),** the nurse should:

1. Weigh the client at the same time each day using the same scale.
   This is a good distractor, since it is a POSSIBILITY. This nursing action is needed to assess adequate nutrition. The purpose of TPN is to provide adequate nutrition. The flow rate must be regulated. If the rate is too fast, hyperosmolar diuresis occurs. If the rate is too slow, inadequate nutrition occurs. By weighing the client daily using the same scale, the nurse is assessing adequate nutrition. Since you have identified the issue, however, you know that you are looking for a common COMPLICATION of TPN. Remember to read all the options before making your decision.

2. Keep accurate records of total intake and total output.
   This is another appropriate nursing action and a POSSIBLE option. Again, the reason to assess intake and output is to assess for adequate nutrition. This option is very similar to option 1. Since both refer to the same idea, however, neither of these options can be the correct answer. Look for the option that is different.

3. Determine the increase or decrease in body weight each day.
   This option is similar to Options 1 and 2 and yet another POSSIBLE option. All of the options so far are concerned with monitoring adequate nutrition. Again, since all three options REFER TO THE SAME IDEA, none of them can be the correct answer. The answer then has to be 4.

4. **Take the client's temperature at least every four hours.**
   This is the only option that addresses the ISSUE in the question, which is monitoring for a common COMPLICATION of TPN. Catheter-related infections are the most common complication of TPN. Options 1, 2, and 3 all address weight and are so similar that there is no reason to prefer one of them over the others. Option 4 is the "different" option and the correct answer. Using the strategy of eliminating similar distractors can improve your understanding of "test-question logic" and increase your score!

DRILL 5

A newly diagnosed adult diabetic is demonstrating of the proper technique for insulin injection. The client draws up the correct dose of insulin using the proper technique, but when ready to inject the needle, hesitates and says, "I'm not sure I can do this." Which response by the nurse would be best initially?

1. "I'll show you again how to inject the needle."
2. "I'll inject the needle for you this time."
3. "You're doing fine so far. Give it a try."
4. "Why are you so nervous? Do you need help?"

ANALYSIS 5

Critical Elements	
Key words:	See bold print
Client:	A newly diagnosed adult diabetic
Issue:	The nurse's initial response to an unsure client demonstrating insulin injection.
Type of Stem:	True response stem

Eliminate Options

A **newly** diagnosed adult diabetic is **demonstrating** of the proper technique for insulin injection. The client draws up the correct dose of insulin using the proper technique, but when ready to inject the needle, hesitates and says, "I'm **not sure** I can do this." Which response by the nurse would be best **initially?**

? 1. "I'll show you again how to inject the needle."
   This response is a POSSIBILITY, since this nursing action may sometimes be appropriate in client teaching. This case scenario states, however, that the client is using the proper technique. This is not the best response because it focuses on the nurse doing the procedure rather than on the client doing the procedure. Remember, the purpose of nursing is to help the client maintain an optimal level of functioning.

? 2. "I'll inject the needle for you this time."
   This is also a POSSIBILITY, but this is similar to option 1 in that the nurse does the procedure.

+ 3. **"You're doing fine so far. Give it a try."**
   This is the correct answer because it focuses on the client being encouraged to do the procedure. This answer is client-centered.

■ 4. "Why are you so nervous? Do you need help?"
"Why" responses are always INCORRECT. This response blocks communication by making the client feel defensive and is not therapeutic because it focuses on the client's nervousness and need for help. Being nervous and unsure is an appropriate feeling for this newly diagnosed adult diabetic. The nurse's response should enhance the client's feelings of competency.

In providing care to a client with COPD, the primary nursing consideration is to:

1. Not overtire the client.
2. Plan adequate rest periods throughout the day.
3. Give only low-flow oxygen.
4. Allow the client to set the pace when walking.

Critical Elements	
Key words:	See bold print
Client:	A client with COPD
Issue:	A primary nursing consideration for a client with COPD
Type of Stem:	True response stem

6 DRILL

6 ANALYSIS

Eliminate Options

In providing care to a client with **COPD,** the **primary** nursing consideration is to:

❓ 1. Not overtire the client.
This is a POSSIBLE answer. A client with COPD needs to avoid activities that produce excessive shortage of breath to preserve existing pulmonary function. You need to continue reading and see if you think that this remains the best option.

❓ 2. Plan adequate rest periods throughout the day.
This is another POSSIBLE answer, but it is similar to option 1. Both refer to rest as the primary nursing consideration in caring for a client with COPD. Since both 1 and 2 present the same idea, neither can be the best answer.

➕ **3. Give only low-flow oxygen.**
This is the correct answer when selecting an option that reflects a nursing PRIORITY. After reading all the options, you will find that

this is the best one. With the diagnosis of COPD, it is IMPORTANT not to remove the hypoxic drive by providing too much oxygen, which can lead to hypoventilation and respiratory insufficiency. This is the only option that refers to the COPD client's special need to maintain low levels of oxygen.

4. Allow the client to set the pace when walking.
   This is a POSSIBLE answer because it would be appropriate. Using the similar distractor test-taking strategy, however, you can eliminate this option because, like options 1 and 2, it is based on the idea of rest.

SIMILAR WORDS

If you don't know the answer, look first for a global response option and try to eliminate similar distractors. If you still cannot choose between the two best options, look for a similar word or phrase used in the stem of the question and in one of the options. If you find a word, feeling, or behavior used in the stem or the case scenario that is repeated in one of the options, that option <u>may</u> be the correct answer. Although looking for similar words is not as reliable as the first two strategies in this chapter, it is helpful when you can't decide on the best answer and the other two strategies cannot be used.

Practice Session: Looking for Similar Words

As you read and answer the following questions, look for an answer that has a similar word or phrase in the stem of the question and in one of the options. First, review the questions by identifying the four critical elements. Then narrow your choices while looking for the option that includes a similar word. After you have answered the question, read the analysis. The **key words** and the **answers** are in **bold** print.

In caring for a client immediately following a cardiac catheterization procedure, which nursing action is appropriate?

1. Applying warm compresses to the puncture site.
2. Assisting with passive range of motion exercises.
3. Monitoring the client for cardiac arrhythmias.
4. Assisting the client into high-Fowler's position.

7 ANALYSIS

Critical Elements	
Key words:	See bold print
Client:	A client following a cardiac catheterization
Issue:	A vital nursing action immediately after a cardiac catheterization
Type of Stem:	True response stem

Eliminate Options

In caring for a client **immediately** following a **cardiac catheterization** procedure, which nursing action is **appropriate?**

■ 1. Apply warm compresses to the puncture site.
This action is UNSAFE! *Because bleeding and hematoma are major complications in the post-procedure period, heat is never applied.*

■ 2. Assist with passive range of motion exercises.
This action is also UNSAFE. *Because of the complication of bleeding, movement is limited in the involved extremity.*

+ **3. Monitor the client for cardiac arrhythmias.**
Irregularities in the heart rate are a VITAL CONCERN *in the post-procedure period. Until the vital signs are stable, the client needs to be closely assessed for arrhythmias. This is the correct answer. Note that the word "cardiac" is also used in the stem.*

■ 4. Assist the client into high Fowler's position.
This is UNSAFE. *This position could obstruct arterial blood flow and lead to formation of a thrombus. The extremity used for the site must be properly aligned and immobilized immediately after the procedure.*

A client sustained a fracture of the tibia and fibula. In providing care for this client, who has a newly applied long-leg cast, which consideration is vital?

1. Elevation of the leg in the cast on a pillow will minimize edema.
2. Healing of a fractured bone requires an extended period of time.
3. A long period of immobility may lead to atrophy of the muscle.
4. Analgesics may be needed for pain associated with the fracture.

ANALYSIS

8

Critical Elements
Key words: See bold print
Client: A client with a fractured tibia and fibula
Issue: A vital consideration when caring for a client with a newly applied cast
Type of Stem: True response stem

Eliminate Options

A client has sustained a fracture of the tibia and fibula. In providing nursing care for this client, who has a **newly applied long-leg cast,** which consideration is **vital?**

+ 1. **Elevation of the leg in the cast on a pillow will minimize edema.**
      When caring for a client with a newly applied cast, it is IMPORTANT *to keep the affected extremity above the level of the heart to reduce swelling. Swelling causes vasoconstriction. Note that the words "leg" and "cast" are repeated in this option.*

? 2. Healing of a fractured bone requires an extended period of time.
      This option might be a POSSIBLE *answer, since this statement correctly states the pathophysiology of a fracture. The issue in the question, however, is a vital action when caring for a client with a newly applied cast. This option does not address the issue of the question.*

? 3. A long period of immobility may lead to atrophy of the muscle.
      Like option 2, this option contains correct information, so it appears to be a POSSIBLE *choice, but it, too, relates to the pathophysiology issue. The focus of the answer has to be a vital nursing consideration.*

+ 4. Analgesics may be needed for pain associated with the fracture.
      This nursing action is NECESSARY *in caring for a fracture. However, the issue is nursing care associated with a* NEWLY APPLIED CAST, *not a fracture, and this is not the most vital consideration. Note that in this question there were two very good answers, only one of which was correct because* IT ALONE ANSWERED THE QUESTION ACTUALLY BEING ASKED. *It is not just coincidence that the one correct answer repeated the words "leg" and "cast."*

Four weeks after a fracture of the tibia and fibula, the nurse notes decreased breath sounds in the lower lobes of both the client's lungs. What is the nurse's best explanation of this change in breath sounds?

1. The client did not take deep breaths while the nurse examined the lower lobes.
2. Because of improper positioning, the client has developed pulmonary edema.
3. Atelectasis caused by immobility resulted in the decreased breath sounds.
4. The client has lowered resistance and has caught a cold from someone else.

9 DRILL

Critical Elements

Key words:	See bold print
Client:	A client with decreased breath sounds
Issue:	Possible rationale for decreased breath sounds four weeks after a fracture
Type of Stem:	True response stem

9 ANALYSIS

Eliminate Options

Four weeks after a fracture of the tibia and fibula the nurse notes **decreased breath sounds** in the lower lobes of both the client's lungs. What is the nurse's best explanation of this change in **breath sounds?**

1. The client did not take deep breaths while the nurse examined the lower lobes.
   This might seem to be a POSSIBLE *explanation, but this option* INTRODUCES NEW INFORMATION *not found in the case scenario. There is no information that the client did not take deep breaths. If you chose this option, you "read into" the question.*

2. Because of improper positioning, the client has developed pulmonary edema.
   Pulmonary edema is USUALLY NOT *a complication caused by immobility from a fracture and would not be the reason for the decreased breath sounds. Pulmonary edema is a complication of heart failure. This option also "read into" the question by adding the improper positioning rationale.*

3. Atelectasis caused by immobility resulted in the decreased breath sounds.

Immobility causes atelectasis, which results in decreased breath sounds. This is the most plausible reason for the decreased breath sounds. This is a fairly difficult question. Note that the words "breath sounds" used in the stem are repeated in this option.

4. The client has lowered resistance and has caught a cold from someone else.

Since there is NO INFORMATION *in the case scenario about the client having a cold, this is not the answer. Be careful not to "read into" the question.*

POINTS TO REMEMBER

1. If you are unable to answer using your nursing knowledge alone, then apply strategies!

2. When more than one option appears correct, look for:
   - A global response
   - Similar distractors that you can eliminate
   - A similar word or phrase used in both the case scenario (or stem) and one of the options

Chapter 5

LEARNING TO ANSWER COMMUNICATION QUESTIONS

Communication is an essential skill in the practice of nursing. The goal of nursing is to help the client attain and maintain an optimal level of functioning. Communication skills are needed to achieve this nursing goal. Since the NCLEX-RN Exam measures your ability to practice safely, communication skills are an integral part of the exam.

> **If you cannot communicate therapeutically, it is difficult to practice safely.**

For this reason, your nursing course exams may also include many communication questions.

Communication skills are recognized as vital at all levels of nursing practice. Today there are communication test questions on every type of certification exam in nursing practice, including the specialty levels. Learning how to answer communication questions will enhance your score on the NCLEX-RN Exam and on other nursing exams.

Students frequently report that there are a great number of questions that refer to the psychiatric clinical setting on NCLEX-RN Exam. Many of these "psych" questions are actually communication questions. According to the NCLEX-RN Exam test plan (see Chapter Nine), the communication thread is a major component of the exam.

The test-taking strategies presented in this chapter will require that you understand the test-taking terminology and techniques presented in Chapters Three and Four. If you have not yet read those chapters, do so before proceeding with Chapter Five. You also should have read the introduction.

Identifying the Client in a Communication Question

You want to start with the test-taking techniques that you learned in Chapter Three. When you identify the critical elements, however, two elements require particular attention. First, you must take care when you identify **the client in the question.** This is not always obvious to the unskilled test-taker, because **the client is not necessarily the person identified with the health problem.**

The client in the question is the person to whom the nurse must respond—and this is almost always someone in the case scenario who has asked the nurse something, or perhaps someone who has done something that affects the nurse. Depending upon the question's case scenario and the stem of the question, the client may be a relative, another client, or even another nurse.

Identifying the Issue

When you identify the issue in the question be prepared for some twists based on the identity of the actual client in the question. **The issue must relate to the client in the question, and the nurse's response must address the client's issue.** Thus, you may get detailed clinical information about a critically ill client whose wife asks the nurse about visiting hours. You must be able to spot the fact that the wife is the client in the question and that the issue then will pertain to her.

Communication Tools and Blocks

Once you have identified the critical elements, particularly the client in the question, the issue, and the type of stem, you need to select your answer. To do this, you need to apply your knowledge of therapeutic communication. The following guidelines summarize the **tools** and **blocks** to therapeutic communication.

Communication tools are mechanisms that **enhance** therapeutic communication. The blocks are responses that **interfere** with communication. Examples of the therapeutic communication tools are shown in the following table.

Therapeutic Communication Tools

Tools	Examples of statements
Being silent	Sitting quietly
Offering self	"Let me sit with you."
Showing empathy	"You are upset."
Focusing	"You say that . . . "
Restatement	"You feel anxious?"
Validation/clarification	"What you are saying is . . . ?"
Giving information	"Your room is 423."
Dealing with the here and now	"At this time, the problem is . . . "

The nurse must be in a therapeutic role. When you answer communication questions, remember that **only options that use therapeutic communication tools can be correct answers (if the question has a true response stem).**

Examples of communication blocks are shown in the table below. After reviewing the tools and blocks, apply these concepts to the questions in the practice session.

Communication Blocks

Blocks	Examples of statements
Giving advice	"If I were you, I would . . . "
Showing approval/disapproval	"You did the right thing."
Using cliches and false reassurances	"Don't worry. It will be all right."
Requesting an explanation	"Why did you do that?"
Devaluing client feelings	"Don't be concerned. It's not a problem."
Being defensive	"Every nurse on this unit is exceptional."
Focusing on inappropriate issues or persons	"Have I said something wrong?"
Placing the client's issues on "hold"	"Talk to your doctor about that."

> A final point to note in answering communication questions is that the nurse must put special emphasis on recognizing and responding to the client's feelings.

Practice Session: Learning to Answer Communication Questions

Read and answer the following questions. When selecting the best response by the nurse, look for the response that enhances communication. Remember to identify the critical elements, especially the client and the issue.

When you have identified the type of stem, narrow your choices. Look for responses by the nurse that use communication tools and responses that address the client's feelings. Remember to apply the three test-taking strategies from Chapter Four, too; these strategies are also extremely useful in communication questions. After you have answered the question, read the analysis. **Key words** and the **correct answers** are in bold print.

DRILL 1

A client is admitted to the hospital for an exploratory laparotomy. The client's daughter says to the nurse, "I wish I could stay with my father, but I need to go home to see how my children are doing. I really hate to leave my father alone at this time." The best nursing response is:

1. "Your father needs opportunities to be independent. This will help him become self-sufficient."
2. "Your father is capable of taking care of himself. Try allowing him more independence."
3. "Stress is not good for your father at this time. Perhaps you could call your children."
4. "You are feeling concern for both your father and your children. Let me know when you are leaving, and I'll stay with him."

ANALYSIS 1

Critical Elements	
Key words:	See bold print
Client:	The daughter
Issue:	A response to the daughter's concerns about needing to leave her father alone
Type of Stem:	True response stem (therapeutic communication)

Eliminate Options

A client is admitted to the hospital for an **exploratory laparotomy**. The **client's daughter says** to the nurse, **"I wish I could stay** with my father, **but I need to go home** to see how my children are doing. **I really hate to leave my father alone** at this time." The **best** nursing response is:

1. "Your father needs opportunities to be independent. This will help him become self-sufficient."
   This is a COMMUNICATION BLOCK because the nurse is giving advice. The daughter is the client in this question, and this response fails to address the client's issue, which is her immediate concern about leaving her father.

2. "Your father is capable of taking care of himself. Try allowing him more independence."
   This is also the communication BLOCK of giving advice. Like option 1, this response does not address the daughter's immediate concern about leaving her father.

3. "Stress is not good for your father at this time. Perhaps you could call your children."
   Like options 1 and 2, this is giving advice and another BLOCK to communication. The answer has to be 4.

4. **"You are feeling concern for both your father and your children. Let me know when you are leaving, and I'll stay with him."**
   This response uses the TOOLS of empathy and offering self. This empathetic response focuses on the client's concerns of the moment, of being both a mother and a daughter, which she has shared with the nurse. The nurse uses the tool of offering self by offering to stay with the father.

An elderly client who is hospitalized for an exploratory laparotomy says to the nurse, "Do you think that the doctor can fix whatever is wrong with me?" Which response by the nurse would be best initially?

1. "That question can only be answered after your surgery."
2. "People your age frequently have problems that can be corrected by surgery."
3. "You need to get more information from your doctor."
4. "You must be worried about what the doctor might find."

ANALYSIS

2

Critical Elements	
Key words:	See bold print
Client:	An elderly client hospitalized for an exploratory laparotomy
Issue:	The client's concerns about possible findings
Type of Stem:	True response stem (therapeutic communication)

Eliminate Options

An **elderly** client who is hospitalized for an **exploratory laparotomy says** to the nurse, "Do you think that the doctor can fix **whatever is wrong with me?**" Which response by the nurse would be best **initially**?

■   1.   "That question can only be answered after your surgery."
The question asks which response is best initially. This is a BLOCK that places the client's feelings on hold. This response might be suitable for a later time, after the nurse has addressed the client's feelings.

■   2.   "People your age frequently have problems that can be corrected by surgery."
This statement may or may not be true; however, the case scenario does not include any information to indicate that the client's suspected health problem is related to age. This response cannot be the answer because it BLOCKS COMMUNICATION by giving false reassurance. It also refers to inappropriate persons ("people your age") and, directly related to that BLOCK, it fails to address the client's feelings.

■   3.   "You need to get more information from your doctor."
In this response the nurse fails to address the client's concerns and feelings. This response is a BLOCK that puts the client's feelings on hold. This response is not therapeutic.

⊞   **4.   "You must be worried about what the doctor might find."**
This is the correct answer, because this response uses two therapeutic communication TOOLS. One is empathy, which is shown by focusing on the client's feelings. The second tool is restatement, a tool that helps the client clarify feelings. Communication theory identifies that the nurse should address the client's feelings, so the "initial response" often will be one that focuses on the client's feelings. After the client's feelings are addressed, information can be more productively communicated.

A 20-day-old infant is recovering from surgery for pyloric stenosis. The mother asks the nurse, "Now that my child has had this surgery, is it likely that pyloric stenosis will cause trouble later?" Which is the most appropriate nursing response?

1. "Why don't you talk to the doctor about your uncertainties regarding your child's future?"
2. "Obstructive manifestations might develop later. If so, go immediately to an emergency room."
3. "Your child will not have manifestations again in childhood, but may have digestive difficulties as an adult."
4. "Recurrence of the obstruction or repetition of the surgical procedure would be unlikely."

Critical Elements	
Key words:	See bold print
Client:	The mother
Issue:	The mother's concern regarding the prognosis for a child with pyloric stenosis
Type of Stem:	True response stem (therapeutic communication)

Eliminate Options

A 20-day-old infant is recovering from surgery for **pyloric stenosis**. The **mother** asks the nurse, "Now that my child has had this surgery, is it likely that pyloric stenosis will cause **trouble later?"** Which is the most **appropriate** nursing response?

1. "Why don't you talk to the doctor about your uncertainties regarding your child's future?"
   This responses uses the BLOCK of placing the client's concerns on hold. The nurse needs to address the issue here and now.

2. "Obstructive manifestations might develop later. If so, go immediately to an emergency room."
   This is a POSSIBILITY. It is true that pyloric stenosis may recur, but this option does not fully answer the mother's question and will increase her fear. Remember, if part of the option is correct and part is incorrect, it makes the whole option wrong.

■ 3. "Your child will not have manifestations again in childhood, but may have digestive difficulties as an adult."
This is too absolute a statement, and it is therefore INACCURATE *information. The nurse cannot say with absolute certainty that the baby will not have manifestations again in childhood. Recurrence is remotely possible.*

✚ **4. "Recurrence of the obstruction or repetition of the surgical procedure would be unlikely."**
This option uses the TOOL *of responding to the mother's concern by providing information that is accurate. A better response might also address the mother's feelings, but no such response is offered with this question. Of all the options, this is the best. You may not like any of the choices, but you cannot skip questions and need to select the best option of those given.*

DRILL 4

A few days after being admitted following a drinking binge, a client with a chronic alcohol problem becomes increasingly agitated and tells the staff that red ants are walking all over the floor and walls. The nurse enters the room and finds the client shouting in a terrified voice, "Get those ants out of my room!" Which nursing response is most therapeutic at this time?

1. "Tell me more about the ants that you see in your room."
2. "I'm sure that the ants you see will not harm you."
3. "I don't see any ants, but you seem very frightened."
4. "I do not see anything. This is part of your illness."

ANALYSIS 4

Critical Elements	
Key words:	See bold print
Client:	A client with a chronic alcohol problem who is hallucinating
Issue:	Response to a hallucinating client who is terrified
Type of Stem:	True response stem (therapeutic communication)

Eliminate Options

A few days after being admitted following a drinking binge, a client with a chronic alcohol problem becomes increasingly **agitated** and tells the staff that **red ants** are walking all over the floor and walls. The nurse enters the room and finds the client shouting in a **terrified** voice, "Get those ants out of my room!" Which of the following comments would be **most therapeutic** at this time?

■ 1. "Tell me more about the ants you see in your room."
This is NOT THERAPEUTIC *because it* BLOCKS *communication by focusing on the ants or the mechanics of the hallucination, rather than on the client's feelings.*

■ 2. "I'm sure that the ants you see will not harm you."
This response uses the BLOCK *of false reassurance—at least the client will perceive it this way! This response also is nontherapeutic because in dealing with hallucinations it is inappropriate to reinforce the hallucination. In this case scenario, the nurse needs to reinforce reality and address the client's feelings.*

+ **3. "I don't see any ants, but you seem very frightened."**
This response PRESENTS REALITY *in an appropriate manner and uses the* COMMUNICATION TOOL *of empathy to address the client's feelings. By saying, "you seem frightened," the nurse acknowledges the client's feelings that have been communicated in his terrified voice. Note that the test-taking strategy of observing a similar word in the case scenario and one of the options can be successfully used here: the words "frightened" and "terrified" are similar.*

? 4. "I do not see anything. This is part of your illness."
This might be a POSSIBILITY, *since this option does present reality; however, this response does not address the client's feelings. Option 3 is better because it uses the tool of empathy.*

After one week of hospitalization, a chronic alcoholic client's son visits and says to the nurse, "I would do anything if my dad would only stop drinking." What would be the initial goal of the nurse's response?

5 DRILL

1. Have the son join a support group like Al-Anon.
2. Reinforce that the family is very supportive of his father.
3. Help the son understand that his father needs to take responsibility for his disease.
4. Help the son explain the problem as he sees it.

Critical Elements	
Key words:	See bold print
Client:	The son of a chronic alcoholic client
Issue:	A son's concern about his chronic alcoholic father.
Type of Stem:	True response stem (therapeutic communication)

5 ANALYSIS

Eliminate Options

After one week of hospitalization, a **chronic alcoholic's son** visits and says to the nurse, "I would do anything if my dad would only stop drinking." What would be the **initial goal** of the nurse's response?

? 1. Have the son join a support group like Al-Anon.
This goal is appropriate and is a POSSIBILITY. However, this question asks for the INITIAL goal regarding the son's present concerns. This option fails to address the son's concern and blocks communication by giving advice.

– 2. Reinforce that the family is very supportive of his father.
This is another BLOCK because it gives false reassurance and does not focus on the son's concerns. This response could also be interpreted as the nurse giving approval, which is nontherapeutic.

? 3. Help the son understand that his father needs to take responsibility for his disease.
This is a POSSIBILITY, however, this question asks about the INITIAL goal. This might be a goal for later.

+ **4. Help the son explain the problem as he sees it.**
This response uses the TOOL of clarification. In order for the son to resolve his problem, the problem needs to be defined. This response helps him clarify his problem. This also reflects the first step of the nursing process, which is assessment. By helping the son to clarify the problem, the nurse is gathering additional information about the son's concern. Before a nursing diagnosis can be made, the nurse must identify and clarify the problem. In Chapter Six you will learn even more about using the nursing process to answer test questions.

DRILL 6

During a lengthy conversation with the nurse about a client's long history of alcoholism, the client becomes obviously tense and uncomfortable. At this time, which of the following remarks by the nurse would be the most appropriate?

1. "What did I say to make you feel uncomfortable?"
2. "Drinking for a long period of time can make anyone feel uncomfortable."
3. "At what point did you begin to feel uncomfortable?"
4. "You need to talk about your long drinking history if you are to recover from your illness."

6 ANALYSIS

Critical Elements

Key words:	See bold print
Client:	A client with a chronic alcohol problem
Issue:	The client's tenseness when talking about his long history of drinking
Type of Stem:	True response stem (therapeutic communication)

Eliminate Options

During a lengthy conversation with the nurse about a client's long history of alcoholism, the client becomes **obviously tense and uncomfortable. At this time,** which of the following remarks would be the **most appropriate**?

1. "What did I say to make you feel uncomfortable?"
   This might appear to be a POSSIBILITY *and it is a good distractor. This option actually* BLOCKS COMMUNICATION *because it focuses on an inappropriate person (the nurse) rather than on the client. The nurse is accepting responsibility for the client's feelings. A therapeutic response focuses on the client rather than on the nurse.*

2. "Drinking for a long period of time can make anyone feel uncomfortable."
   This response is a BLOCK *that devalues the client's feelings. It's like saying, "We all get depressed."*

3. **"At what point did you begin to feel uncomfortable?"**
   This response uses the TOOL *of clarification. The nurse needs to gather more information about the client's feelings concerning his long history of alcoholism, in order to assess the problem. This response also addresses the client's feelings, using the tool of empathy.*

4. "You need to talk about your long drinking history if you are to recover from your illness."
   This is the BLOCK *of giving advice. Also note that the test-taking strategy of eliminating similar options would be helpful here. Options 1, 2, and 4 are similar in that they all focus on the long history of drinking, so none of those options can be the answer.*

Soon after being admitted to a rehabilitation unit, a client with a chronic alcohol problem says to the nurse, "I don't really need to be here. My wife and family make me drink. My wife spends all my money. My son just had an accident with his car that cost me a fortune in repairs." The most appropriate nursing response at this time is:

7 DRILL

1. "Tell me more about your wife spending all your money."
2. "How did your son's car accident cost you money?"
3. "It sounds like you have financial difficulties."
4. "Tell me more about your concern about being here."

ANALYSIS 7

Critical Elements	
Key words:	See bold print
Client:	A client with a chronic alcohol problem
Issue:	The client's tenseness when talking about his long history of drinking
Type of Stem:	True response stem (therapeutic communication)

Eliminate Options

Soon after being admitted to a rehabilitation unit, a client with a **chronic alcohol problem** says to the nurse, "**I don't really need to be here.** My wife and family make me drink. My wife spends all my money. My son just had an accident with his car that cost me a fortune in repairs." The **most appropriate** nursing response **at this time** is:

■ 1. "Tell me more about your wife spending all your money."
   This is a BLOCK because it focuses on the client's wife and money rather than on the client and his problem. This response addresses an inappropriate issue and an inappropriate person.

■ 2. "How did your son's car accident cost you money?"
   This response also focuses on an INAPPROPRIATE ISSUE. It addresses the client's child and money problems and not his denial.

■ 3. "It sounds like you have financial difficulties."
   This is a good distractor because it begins with clarification words ("it sounds like"), but it is NONTHERAPEUTIC because it focuses on money as the issue rather than on the client's denial. Note that options 1, 2, and 3 all focus on money or finances. Option 4 is the different one.

✚ **4. "Tell me more about your concern about being here."**
   This response is the answer because it uses the TOOL of empathy, focusing on the client's feelings. Also, note that this response is the only response that addresses the client's denial, which is the issue in the question.

Chapter 6

LEARNING TO ANSWER QUESTIONS THAT SELECT PRIORITIES

Recognizing Priority-Setting Questions

The NCLEX-RN Exam test plan focuses on the application and analysis of nursing knowledge. Consequently, your nursing course exams as well as the NCLEX use test questions that require decision making, such as those that involve selecting priorities. These questions are difficult.

Here are some examples of the stems found in questions that select priorities:

- What is the nurse's **initial** response?

- What is the **essential** nursing action?

- What is a **vital** consideration in planning the client's nursing care?

- The nurse would give **immediate** attention to which of the following questions?

- What nursing action receives the **highest** priority?

- Which response demonstrates the **best** nursing judgment?

- Which information is **most** important?

Four Prioritizing Guidelines for Nursing Exams

The following table presents quick summaries of four different guidelines you can use in questions that ask you to select priorities.

Guidelines Used to Select Priorities

Maslow's hierarchy of needs
Physiological needs come first. When no physiological needs are identified, safety needs receive priority.

Nursing process
Assessment comes first.

Communication theory
Focus on feelings first.

Teaching/learning theory
Focus on motivation first.

Practice Session: Questions that Require Setting Priorities

Each of the following questions uses one of the priority-setting guidelines mentioned in the table above. As you read each question, try to determine which of the four guidelines provides the rationale for the correct answer for each question. To do this, you will need to read all of the options as well as the case scenario and stem.

Be sure to use all your new test-taking skills when answering these priority-setting questions. First, identify the four critical elements. Then narrow your choices, keeping in mind the guidelines for selecting priorities. If you are unsure of the answer, try using one of the test-taking strategies.

After you have answered the question, read the analysis. Note that the **key words** and the **correct answer** are in **bold** print.

A client is hospitalized with chronic obstructive pulmonary disease (COPD). Oxygen per nasal cannula at 2 liters per minute is initiated. When the nurse made an assessment at 3:00 p.m., the client appeared to have made a good adjustment to hospitalization. At 5:00 p.m., the nurse found the oxygen cannula on the floor. The client was angry and said, "It's about time you got here. Where am I? Where is my breakfast?" The nurse should give immediate consideration to which of the following questions?

1. Has the oxygen cannula been off long enough to cause hypoxia?
2. Is the client's anger related to being hospitalized?
3. Does the client need a clock in the room to keep track of time?
4. Is the client accustomed to eating dinner very early in the day?

Critical Elements

Key words:	See bold print
Client:	A client with COPD who suddenly displays confused behavior
Issue:	Immediate consideration of the nursing priority in caring for the client at this time
Type of Stem:	True response stem

Eliminate Options

A client is hospitalized with **chronic obstructive pulmonary disease (COPD).** Oxygen per nasal cannula at 2 liters per minute is initiated. When the nurse made an assessment at 3:00 p.m., the client appeared to have made a good adjustment to hospitalization. At 5:00 p.m., the nurse found the **oxygen cannula on the floor.** The client was angry and said, "It's about time you got here. **Where am I? Where is my breakfast?"** The nurse should give **immediate** consideration to which of the following questions?

1. **Has the oxygen cannula been off long enough to cause hypoxia?** *This question is a* HIGH PRIORITY *because it focuses on an immediate physiological need. A low flow of oxygen is necessary to maintain the hypoxic drive for a client with COPD. Due to the confused behavior and lack of oxygen for a period of time, the client may be exhibiting signs of acute respiratory insufficiency. Here the priority is a life-threatening situation, and* MASLOW'S HIERARCHY OF NEEDS *is the priority-setting guideline to be used. You also may have noticed that the key words "oxygen cannula" appeared only in this option!*

■   2. Is the client's anger related to being hospitalized?
        *This is a LOW PRIORITY response because it addresses a PSYCHO-
        LOGICAL consideration as an explanation for the client's behavior.
        It must first be determined whether or not the behavior may be due
        to a PHYSIOLOGICAL need. Note that the case scenario also states
        that the client appeared to have made a good adjustment to hospi-
        talization.*

■   3. Does the client need a clock in the room to keep track of time?
        *This is another LOW PRIORITY response. This option is similar to
        option 2 in that it suggests a psychological rationale for the client's
        behavior. This reason would be explored only after clarifying that
        the behavior was not due to a respiratory insufficiency.*

■   4. Is the client accustomed to eating dinner very early in the day?
        *This is another LOW PRIORITY response. This option is similar to
        option 3 because it focuses on the issue of time of day. Using
        Maslow's hierarchy of needs as a guideline, physiological needs re-
        ceive priority. Note that you can also use the test-taking strategy of
        eliminating similar distractors in this question. Since options 2, 3,
        and 4 all focus on psychological considerations, look for the option
        that is different.*

DRILL 2

A client hospitalized with COPD has just recovered from an episode of
confused behavior as a result of respiratory insufficiency. At dinner time,
the nurse assists the client with the oxygen cannula and raises the head of
the bed to high-Fowler's position. Then the nurse places the dinner tray
on the over-bed table and prepares the dinner according to the client's
preference. Which nursing action is most essential before leaving the
room?

1. Ask the client if further assistance is needed with the meal.
2. Assist the client with menu selections for the following day.
3. Tell the client that the nurse will return in about 30 minutes.
4. Place the call bell where the client can easily reach it.

ANALYSIS 2

Critical Elements	
Key words:	See bold print
Client:	A client with COPD who has experienced hypoxia and confusion
Issue:	The priority nursing action when leaving the client's room
Type of Stem:	True response stem

Eliminate Options

A client hospitalized with **COPD** has **just recovered** from an episode of **confused behavior** as a result of **respiratory insufficiency.** At dinner time, the nurse assists the client with the oxygen cannula and raises the head of the bed to high-Fowler's position. Then the nurse places the dinner tray on the over-bed table and prepares the dinner according to the client's preference. Which nursing action is **most essential before leaving the room?**

[?] 1. Ask the client if further assistance is needed with the meal.
This option is a POSSIBILITY because this is an appropriate nursing action; however, it might not be a priority. Remember to review all the other options before making a decision. Which priority-setting guideline is used in this question?

[?] 2. Assist the client with menu selections for the following day.
This nursing action would be appropriate, so it might be a POSSIBILITY. However, like option 1, this option is concerned with the client's meals. Look for a nursing action that would receive higher priority.

[–] 3. Tell the client that the nurse will return in about 30 minutes.
This action is INAPPROPRIATE. Since the client was confused and hypoxic, his condition would warrant more frequent checks. This action will not provide for the client's safety.

[+] **4. Place the call bell where the client can easily reach it.**
This is a HIGH-PRIORITY nursing action because it addresses the client's need for a safe environment. Because of the confused behavior and restrictions with mobility, providing a safe environment in which the client has access to a call bell is a priority. Here Maslow's hierarchy of needs is used as a guideline. If a physiological need is not the issue, then SAFETY needs receive priority.

A client hospitalized with COPD is receiving oxygen by nasal cannula. At 5:00 p.m. the oxygen cannula was found on the floor, and the nurse assisted the client with the oxygen cannula and raised the head of the bed to high-Fowler's position. At 8:45 p.m., the client reports feeling short of breath and requests to change position. In addition to repositioning the client, the nurse should give highest priority to which nursing action?

1. Put the client on 15-minute checks.
2. Call the physician to report the shortness of breath.
3. Observe the rate, depth, and character of the client's respirations.
4. Help the client relax by giving a back rub.

ANALYSIS 3

Critical Elements	
Key words:	See bold print
Client:	A client with COPD
Issue:	Shortness of breath
Type of Stem:	True response stem

Eliminate Options

A client hospitalized with **COPD** is receiving oxygen by nasal cannula. At 5:00 p.m. **the oxygen cannula was found on the floor,** and the nurse assisted the client with the oxygen cannula and raised the head of the bed to high-Fowler's position. At 8:45 p.m., the client reports feeling **short of breath** and requests to change position. In addition to repositioning the client, the nurse should give **highest priority** to which nursing action?

[?] 1. Put the client on 15-minute checks.
This is a POSSIBILITY. *Any client with a breathing problem must be monitored closely because this could be a medical emergency. However, this is an* IMPLEMENTATION *action. Checking the client every 15 minutes implies that the nurse has diagnosed that the shortness of breath is not a medical emergency. Which priority-setting guideline will you use in this question?*

[?] 2. Call the physician to report the shortness of breath.
This is another POSSIBILITY, *but it, too, is an implementation action. Reporting to the physician implies that the nurse has diagnosed that this is a medical emergency. The question, however, gives no information about whether this is a medical emergency. What should the nurse do at this time?*

[+] **3. Observe the rate, depth, and character of the client's respirations.**
This assessment action receives HIGHEST PRIORITY *in this case scenario. Before you call the physician, an* ASSESSMENT *is needed of the client's respiratory status. This question uses the* NURSING PROCESS *as a guideline: before any nursing action is implemented, an assessment is needed. You will see that the nursing process is not just a prioritizing guideline in Chapter Seven but, for now, remember that it can be extremely useful when you are faced with a priority-setting question.*

4. Help the client relax by giving a back rub.
This implementation action may be appropriate, but it addresses a psychological need and would therefore have a low priority. It also does not indicate that the nurse has assessed the client to determine that a back rub would be appropriate.

An client with COPD is admitted to the hospital. While bathing, the client says, "I don't know why I have to be here. Everything around here is a constant reminder of how sick I am." Which nursing response is best initially?

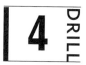

1. "Don't worry. Your doctor will let you go home in a few days."
2. "Why don't you like the hospital? Is it something I said or did?"
3. "If I were you, I'd go to sleep. Tomorrow you will feel better."
4. "Tell me more about what you don't like in the hospital."

Critical Elements	
Key words:	See bold print
Client:	A client with COPD
Issue:	Client's feelings about illness and hospitalization
Type of Stem:	True response stem

Eliminate Options

An client with COPD is admitted to the hospital. While bathing the client states, **"I don't know why I have to be here.** Everything around here is a constant reminder of **how sick I am."** Which nursing response is **best initially**?

1. "Don't worry. Your doctor will let you go home in a few days."
This response is NONTHERAPEUTIC because it uses false reassurance and demeans the client's feelings.

2. "Why don't you like the hospital? Is it something I said or did?"
This "why" question BLOCKS COMMUNICATION by putting the client on the defensive. "Why" questions are not therapeutic because they make clients feel like they is being interrogated. The second part of the nurse's response also blocks communication by focusing on an inappropriate person (the nurse).

■ 3. "If I were you, I'd go to sleep. Tomorrow you will feel better."
This response is a BLOCK *because the nurse is giving advice and giving false reassurance.*

+ **4. "Tell me more about what you don't like in the hospital."**
This THERAPEUTIC *response uses* COMMUNICATION THEORY *and addresses the client's feelings and concerns. This is the best initial response because communication theory indicates that the nurse should first address the client's feelings. The nurse uses the communication tool of clarification to encourage the client to discuss and explore concerns about being hospitalized.*

DRILL 5

In preparing an elderly client with COPD to be discharged, the nurse is teaching the client about the correct position for postural drainage. To achieve success in this teaching program, which information about the client is most important? The:

1. Type of bed the client will be using at home for the procedure.
2. Amount of time required for the client to change positions.
3. Client's goal concerning the ability to be self-sufficient.
4. Client's ability to move about without assistance from others.

ANALYSIS 5

Critical Elements	
Key words:	See bold print
Client:	An elderly client with COPD
Issue:	Critical information about the client needed for
	planning successful discharge teaching program
Type of Stem:	True response stem

Eliminate Options

In preparing **an elderly client with COPD** to be **discharged,** the nurse is teaching the client about the correct position for postural drainage. To achieve success in this **teaching program,** which information about the client is **most important?** The:

?   1. Type of bed the client will be using at home for the procedure.
This might be a POSSIBILITY. *Maintaining pulmonary function by effective postural drainage is important. A mechanical bed that facilitates postural drainage is very important, however, you should read all the other options to see if there is a more important consideration.*

?   2. Amount of time required for the client to change positions.
This option is another POSSIBILITY. *Options 1 and 2 both concern very specific information, however, so you want to start looking for a more global option that fits the criterion. Continue reading.*

+   **3. Client's goal concerning the ability to be self-sufficient.**
According to TEACHING/LEARNING THEORY, *the client's motivations and goals are a* PRIMARY CONCERN *for success in any teaching program. If a client is not motivated or goal directed, a discharge teaching program is not effective. Note that this option is also very global, in comparison to options 1, 2 and 4.*

?   4. Client's ability to move about without assistance from others.
This option is another good POSSIBILITY. *When selecting between options 3 and 4, however, 3 is the better choice because the client must first be motivated for the teaching to be effective. The focus of this question is to measure success in a teaching program—not the effectiveness of postural drainage.*

NOTES

Chapter 7

LEARNING TO ANSWER QUESTIONS THAT INVOLVE THE NURSING PROCESS

Your nursing course exams, as well as the NCLEX-RN Exam, incorporate the nursing process as an integral part of the test plan because this is **the method by which one applies nursing knowledge** in the practice of nursing. In Chapter Six, you were introduced to using the nursing process as a prioritizing guideline. In this chapter you will gain additional experience with the prioritizing aspect of the nursing process and you will practice questions designed to test your ability to apply and understand it as well.

> **Nursing course exams and the NCLEX-RN Exam test plan incorporate all five categories or phases of the nursing process: assessment, analysis, planning, implementation, and evaluation.**

For this reason, when preparing for any nursing exam, it is beneficial to practice answering test questions that involve the nursing process. This is especially true for the NCLEX-RN: on this exam, the questions are equally distributed among the five categories.

In this chapter, test questions are presented that reflect each of the five categories of the nursing process. Follow along to review the specific nursing behaviors associated with each category of the nursing process.

ASSESSMENT

Nursing Behaviors Associated with the Assessment Phase of the Nursing Process

---

- Gathering objective and subjective data
- Identifying manifestations
- Evaluating environments
- Identifying the nurse's reaction
- Verifying data
- Communicating information

When answering questions that focus on the assessment process, keep in mind the following:

- Terms such as "observe," "monitor," "check," "obtain information" or "find out" all refer to the assessment process.

- Remember to **assess first,** before planning or implementing nursing care.

- When assessing, be sure to focus on the **issue** of the question. For example, is it a drug, a disorder, or an early manifestation of a complication?

Practice Session: Learning to Answer Assessment Questions

Read and answer the following assessment questions. Remember to identify the critical elements. When you know the type of stem and the issue, make a decision about each option as you read it by using the selection procedure, keeping in mind the nursing behaviors included in assessment. After you have answered the question, read the analysis. The **key words** and the **correct answer** are in **bold** print.

The practice sessions on the other four categories of the nursing process require similar problem-solving and test-taking methods. (**Always** identify the critical elements and use your test-taking strategies!)

A client is returning from the recovery room to the surgical unit following abdominal surgery. Upon the client's arrival in the care unit, which parameter would be the initial focus of the nurse's assessment?

1. Urine output.
2. Vital signs.
3. Pain in the incision.
4. Status of the dressing.

Critical Elements	
Key words:	See bold print
Client:	A client returning after abdominal surgery
Issue:	Initial focus of postoperative nursing assessment
Type of Stem:	True response stem

Eliminate Options

A client is returning from the recovery room to the surgical unit **following abdominal surgery**. Upon the client's arrival in the care unit, which parameter would be the **initial** focus of the nurse's **assessment?**

? 1. Urine output.

This is a POSSIBILITY, since postoperative assessment of urine output is necessary to measure renal, circulatory, and genitourinary function. However, this would not be the initial focus for postoperative assessment. When answering questions that require prioritizing, remember to read all options before selecting the answer.

+ **2. Vital signs.**

This is the INITIAL FOCUS of your assessment. At this time, the nurse needs to gather objective data about the client's condition. This is a critical situation in which it is necessary to implement the ABC guideline. First, the airway and breathing are monitored by observing the rate of respirations. Next, the circulation is assessed by monitoring the pulse rate and the blood pressure.

? 3. Pain in the incision.

This is an appropriate assessment and a POSSIBLE option, but not the focus of your initial assessment. It is necessary to manage and monitor postoperative pain since the greatest postoperative pain occurs during the first 12 to 36 hours. Potent drugs may depress the respiratory rate and increase tracheal secretions. Management of pain is necessary for client comfort and prevention of postoperative atelectasis and pneumonia. However, this is not the highest priority.

? 4. Status of the dressing.
This is another POSSIBILITY, since it is necessary to observe the dressing for amount, type, odor, and consistency of the drainage. Any drainage is marked and noted on the dressing. This is another important assessment, but it is not the initial focus.

DRILL 2

The nurse caring for a client who is receiving an intravenous infusion has been monitoring the IV site for signs of infiltration. In assessing an IV site that has become infiltrated, the nurse knows that which finding is unexpected?

1. The infusion rate slows or stops while the tubing is not kinked.
2. The area around the injection site feels warm to the touch.
3. Swelling, hardness, or pain is found around the needle site.
4. Blood fails to return in the tubing when the bottle is lowered.

ANALYSIS 2

Critical Elements	
Key words:	See bold print
Client:	A client receiving IV infusion
Issue:	Signs of infiltration
Type of Stem:	False response stem

Eliminate Options

The nurse caring for a client who is receiving an **intravenous infusion** has been monitoring the IV site for signs of infiltration. In **assessing** an IV site that has become **infiltrated**, the nurse knows that which finding is **unexpected**?

■ 1. The infusion rate slows or stops while the tubing is not kinked.
This finding is INDICATIVE of an infiltration. You are looking for a finding that is UNEXPECTED in an infiltration. When infiltration occurs, the IV fluid enters the subcutaneous space and the flow of the IV fluid decreases or may even stop. The area around the venipuncture site swells from the tissue fluid. Note that this assessment question has a false response stem!

+ **2. The area around the injection site feels warm to the touch.**
Since this false response stem asks for a finding that is NOT EX-PECTED in an infiltration, this is the correct response. IV fluid is cool, which causes the area around the venipuncture site to be cool. A warm skin temperature indicates phlebitis, not an infiltration.

– 3. Swelling, hardness, or pain located around the needle site.
This is an EXPECTED FINDING when an infiltration occurs. Swelling occurs as the fluid seeps into the tissue spaces. This is objective data that the nurse would observe when assessing an infiltration of an IV. As the edema continues, the discomfort and pain increase.

– 4. Blood fails to return in the tubing when the bottle is lowered.
This is another EXPECTED FINDING with an infiltration. If the IV is patent when the bottle is lowered, the blood in the vein will flow into the IV tubing. When the needle is dislodged from the vein, blood will fail to return in the tubing when the bottle is lowered. This is not the answer, because the question has a false response stem.

A client is eight hours postoperative after a transurethral resection of the prostate gland (TURP). Which nursing assessment would be an early indication of a postoperative complication?

1. Pain in the operative site.
2. Pulse rate of 88.
3. Output of bloody urine.
4. Oral temperature of 101.8° F.

Critical Elements	
Key words:	See bold print
Client:	A client eight hours post TURP
Issue:	An early indication of a postoperative complication
Type of Stem:	True response stem

Eliminate Options

A client is eight hours postoperative after a transurethral resection of the prostate gland (TURP). Which nursing **assessment** would be an **early** indication of a **postoperative complication**?

?   1. Pain in the operative site.
This is a POSSIBILITY; however, pain is expected and normal after an operation. Pain is one of the earliest manifestations a client experiences when returning to consciousness. The issue of the question, however, is an early indication of a complication. Pain in the operative site does not indicate a complication.

–   2. Pulse rate of 88.
This NORMAL finding is not a sign of a complication.

?   3. Output of bloody urine.
This is a POSSIBILITY; however, bloody urine is expected post TURP. As healing progresses, the urine turns to a pink, then light straw color, and is then free of clots. Since this assessment reflects a normal postoperative course, it does not relate to the issue of the question, which is an early indication of a complication.

+   4. **Oral temperature of 101.8° F.**
A temperature of 101.8° F eight hours postoperatively is considered an early indication of a postoperative complication. A temperature that occurs within the first 24 hours after surgery is usually caused by a pulmonary problem, such as atelectasis. Having the client cough and breathe deeply helps expel mucus plugs that cause collapse of the pulmonary alveoli. This option is the only manifestation that is unexpected in a normal postoperative course and is an early indication of a postoperative problem.

ANALYSIS

Nursing Behaviors Associated with the Analysis Phase of the Nursing Process
• Interpreting data • Validating data • Organizing related data • Identifying a nursing diagnosis

Questions that focus on the analysis phase of the nursing process are the most difficult questions. They require an understanding of the principles of pathophysiology, pharmacokinetics, and psychopathology, as well as growth and development. When answering an analysis question, be sure you have correctly identified the issue of the question. For example, the rationale for bed rest for a client with pneumonia is different than that for a client with a myocardial infarction.

Practice Session: Learning to Answer Analysis Questions

A client, is admitted with a history of myoma of the uterus. She is to have a hysterectomy. In preparing a preoperative teaching plan, the nurse would give top priority to:

1. Active range of motion exercises.
2. A rationale for various tubes, IV's, etc.
3. The need to record vital signs frequently.
4. Coughing and deep breathing exercises.

Critical Elements	
Key words:	See bold print
Client:	A 64-year-old client scheduled for a hysterectomy
Issue:	Preoperative teaching
Type of Stem:	True response stem

Eliminate Options

A client, is admitted with a history of myoma of the uterus. She is to have a **hysterectomy.** In preparing a **preoperative** teaching plan, the nurse would give **top priority** to:

1. Active range of motion exercises.
   This is INAPPROPRIATE, since passive, not active, range of motion exercises are usually performed after surgery.

2. A rationale for various tubes, IV's, etc.
   This is a POSSIBILITY, since knowing the reason for procedures and equipment helps to relieve anxiety. When selecting the highest priority, however, be sure to review all options before making your selection.

■ 3. The need to record vital signs frequently.
This is INAPPROPRIATE, *since this is a nursing priority, not a teaching priority for the client.*

➕ **4. Coughing and deep breathing exercises.**
Teaching skills that involve the client's cooperation in the postoperative period are a PRIORITY *preoperatively. Pulmonary complications are a common postoperative complication. Teaching the client to cough and deep breathe properly helps eliminate mucous plugs that cause atelectasis in the postoperative period.*

DRILL 5

The nurse is performing a developmental evaluation of a two-year-old child. Which observation would the nurse consider a good indicator of normal development?

1. Having command of a vocabulary of six words.
2. The ability to walk up and down stairs without help.
3. The ability to dress and undress.
4. The ability to point at something that is wanted.

ANALYSIS 5

Critical Elements	
Key words:	See bold print
Client:	A two-year-old child
Issue:	A normal developmental characteristic
Type of Stem:	True response stem

Eliminate Options

The nurse is performing a developmental evaluation of a **two-year-old** child. Which observation would the nurse consider a **good indicator of normal development**?

■ 1. Having command of a vocabulary of six words.
This is NOT NORMAL. *A two-year-old has a vocabulary of about 200 to 300 words. An 18-month-old child has a vocabulary of about 10 words.*

➕ **2. The ability to walk up and down stairs without help.**
This is a good indicator of NORMAL *psychomotor development. An 18-month-old walks upstairs, but a two-year-old manages to walk up and down the stairs.*

■ 3. The ability to dress and undress.
This is an INAPPROPRIATE *expectation for a two-year-old. This describes an older child of about three to four years old. A two to three year old is only able to* UNDRESS, *not dress.*

■ 4. The ability to point at something that is wanted.
This is NOT NORMAL *communication ability for a two-year old. This describes a one-year-old infant. Because of increased language ability, a normal two year old does not need to point.*

A client had a cholecystectomy this morning and returned to the unit eight hours ago. The client's temperature is now 102.4° F and the dressing is dry and intact. The client has not yet been out of bed, has complained of incisional pain and was medicated with meperidine (Demerol) about 30 minutes ago. What should the nurse do first?

1. Give the client acetaminophen (Tylenol) 650 mg P.O. immediately.
2. Report the elevated temperature to the physician.
3. Do a physical assessment of the client's chest.
4. Send a urine specimen to the lab for culture.

Critical Elements	
Key words:	See bold print
Client:	A client eight hours post cholecystectomy
Issue:	Signs of postoperative complications
Type of Stem:	True response stem

Eliminate Options

A client had a **cholecystectomy** this morning and returned to the unit **eight hours ago**. The client's temperature is now **102.4° F** and the **dressing is dry and intact**. The client has **not yet been out of bed,** has complained of **incisional pain** and was medicated with **meperidine (Demerol)** about **30 minutes ago**. What should the nurse **do first**?

❓ 1. Give the client acetaminophen (Tylenol) 650 mg P.O. immediately.
This is a POSSIBILITY, *since the client does have an elevated temperature that needs to be medicated—but is this the priority at this time? What is the issue in this question? What should the nurse do first? Review the other options to see if another action would receive higher priority.*

?   2. Report the elevated temperature to the physician.
This is a POSSIBILITY; certainly, this temperature needs to be reported. Again, look at all the answers to see if another action would take priority.

+   **3. Do a physical assessment of the client's chest.**
This action is the NURSING PRIORITY in this case scenario, because the elevated temperature is a sign of a possible postoperative COMPLICATION in a client who was immobilized by surgery and medication. Eight hours after surgery, the nurse assessed the client to have an elevated temperature. A temperature in the first 24-hour period is usually due to a pulmonary problem. At this time, more data needs to be collected about the client's lungs. First, a physical assessment of the chest is needed. After this assessment is made, information about the elevated temperature and the physical chest assessment needs to be reported to the physician. This question requires an ANALYSIS of the assessment data and priority setting.

?   4. Send a urine specimen to the lab for culture.
This is another POSSIBILITY; however, a urine infection would occur about 48 hours after surgery and is unlikely at this time. In addition, note that this option represents a MEDICAL ACTION and not a nursing action. Avoid actions that are not within the domain of nursing!

DRILL 7

An 18-month-old toddler has just undergone a craniotomy. In the immediate postoperative period, the nurse would give top priority to which manifestation?

1. Blood pressure of 80/60.
2. Change in the level of consciousness.
3. Depressed fontanelle.
4. Pulse rate of 130.

ANALYSIS 7

Critical Elements	
Key words:	See bold print
Client:	A toddler in the immediate postcraniotomy period
Issue:	Signs of postoperative complications
Type of Stem:	True response stem

Eliminate Options

An **18-month-old toddler** has just undergone a **craniotomy.** In the **immediate postoperative** period the nurse would give **top priority** to which **manifestation?**

◼ 1. Blood pressure of 80/60.
This is a NORMAL *value for the blood pressure of an 18-month-old. Be sure to know age-appropriate vital signs!*

✚ **2. Change in the level of consciousness.**
This is the initial manifestation of increased intracranial pressure and could signal a LIFE-THREATENING COMPLICATION *after a craniotomy. Behavior changes such as restlessness, fatigue, lethargy, stupor, and coma occur as the pressure increases. This finding necessitates immediate action by the nurse.*

◼ 3. Depressed fontanelle.
This is NOT A PRIORITY. *A depressed fontanelle is evident in fluid loss and dehydration.*

◼ 4. Pulse rate of 130.
This is a NORMAL *pulse rate for a toddler.*

PLANNING

Nursing Behaviors Associated with the Planning Phase of the Nursing Process
• Developing and modifying nursing care plans • Cooperating with other health personnel for delivery of client care • Recording relevant information

When answering questions that focus on the planning process, keep in mind the following:

- The answer involves something that is included in the *nursing* care plan, rather than in the *medical* plan. This exam is about nursing, so focus on the nursing action rather than on the medical action.

- When planning specific care, highlight the issue of the question.

Practice Session: Learning to Answer Planning Questions

DRILL 8

A client has had an upper gastrointestinal fibroscopy. Which nursing measure must the nurse plan to include in the immediate post-procedure care?

1. Connect the nasogastric tube to gravity drainage.
2. Keep the client flat in bed for two hours.
3. Have the client cough and deep breathe every two hours.
4. Instruct visitors not to give ice chips to the client.

ANALYSIS 8

Critical Elements	
Key words:	See bold print
Client:	A client post upper GI fibroscopy
Issue:	A necessary postoperative measure to include in the postoperative nursing care plan
Type of Stem:	True response stem

Eliminate Options

A client has had an **upper gastrointestinal fibroscopy.** Which nursing measure **must** the nurse plan to include in the **immediate post-procedure care**?

■ 1. Connect the nasogastric tube to gravity drainage.
This is INAPPROPRIATE. *This procedure does not involve a nasogastric tube. In this procedure, a lighted endoscope is inserted to visualize the gastric mucosa.*

■ 2. Keep the client flat in bed for two hours.
This also is INAPPROPRIATE, *since the client is able to freely move around after the procedure. Before the procedure, a sedative or a tranquilizer is given for relaxation. The client is fully awake during the procedure.*

■ 3. Have the client cough and deep breathe every two hours.
THIS IS UNNECESSARY AND INAPPROPRIATE, *since this procedure does not involve a general anesthetic.*

+ **4. Instruct visitors not to give ice chips to the client.**
Of the four options given, this is the only APPROPRIATE *nursing measure. A topical anesthetic is used to prevent the client from gagging during the procedure, so it is necessary to check that the gag reflex has returned before offering food or fluids. The gag reflex is checked by tickling the back of the throat with a tongue depressor. The gag reflex should return approximately two hours after the procedure.*

After the repair of a cleft palate, a client is stable and is being transferred to the pediatric unit from the recovery room. Which nursing measure would be inappropriate for the nurse to include in the plan of care for this client?

9 DRILL

1. Keep the client under close observation for early manifestations of respiratory obstruction.
2. Position the client on the abdomen or side to provide adequate drainage.
3. Use frequent suctioning of the oropharynx to clear secretions.
4. Use arm restraints to prevent the client's hands or other objects from getting into the mouth.

Critical Elements
Key words: See bold print
Client: A child returning following surgical repair of cleft palate
Issue: Postoperative nursing plan of care
Type of Stem: False response stem

9 ANALYSIS

Eliminate Options

After the **repair of a cleft palate,** the client is stable and is being transferred to the pediatric unit from the recovery room. Which nursing measure would be **inappropriate** for the nurse to include in the **plan of care** for this client?

– 1. Keep the client under close observation for early manifestations of respiratory obstruction.
This nursing measure is APPROPRIATE. *After repair of a cleft palate, the child needs to adjust to breathing with a closed palate. Also, increased mucus secretions may cause obstruction. Remember, this question has a false response stem.*

■   2. Positioning the client on the abdomen or side to provide adequate drainage.
This is another APPROPRIATE *postoperative nursing measure. Since the suture line is inside the mouth, positioning on the abdomen or side is necessary to promote drainage.*

✚   **3. Use frequent suctioning of the oropharynx to clear secretions.**
This nursing measure is CONTRAINDICATED, *so this is the answer to this false response stem. Suctioning may injure the suture line. The suture line needs to be protected from injury and infection. Meticulous care is given to drain secretions by positioning, and to irrigate the suture line to prevent infection.*

■   4. Use of arm restraints to prevent the client's hands or other objects from getting into the mouth.
This nursing measure is APPROPRIATE *for this client postoperatively. Restraints are used to prevent injury to the suture line.*

DRILL 10

In preparing to teach a hypertensive female client to care for her health problem, the nurse knows that which goal is inappropriate? The client will:

1. Exercise moderately each day.
2. Maintain weight appropriate for height.
3. Discontinue use of birth control pills.
4. Eliminate sodium from her diet.

ANALYSIS 10

Critical Elements	
Key words:	See bold print
Client:	A female hypertensive client
Issue:	Goal for client teaching
Type of Stem:	False response stem

Eliminate Options

In preparing to **teach** a **hypertensive female** client to care for her health problem, the nurse knows that which **goal** is **inappropriate**? The client will:

■ 1. Exercise moderately each day.
   This goal is APPROPRIATE. There is evidence that hypertension occurs among people who are in poor physical condition. Remember, the answer must be an INAPPROPRIATE *goal.*

■ 2. Maintain weight appropriate for height.
   This is another APPROPRIATE goal. Excessive body weight causes an increase in arterial pressure. Control of body weight is helpful in reducing hypertension.

■ 3. Discontinue use of birth control pills.
   This also is APPROPRIATE. Birth control pills and estrogen supplements increase the risk of hypertension.

⊞ **4. Eliminate sodium from her diet.**
   This INAPPROPRIATE *goal is the answer. The complete elimination of sodium from the diet is neither possible nor desirable. It is recommended instead to limit and restrict the amount of sodium in the diet.*

IMPLEMENTATION

Nursing Behaviors Associated with the Implementation Phase of the Nursing Process

- Performing or assisting in performing activities of daily living
- Counseling and teaching clients or families
- Using therapeutic communication skills
- Providing care to achieve therapeutic goals
- Providing care to optimize achievement of health goals by the client
- Supervising and checking the work of the staff

When answering questions that focus on the implementation process, keep in mind the following:

- This kind of question asks the nurse to explain, teach, instruct, or respond to the client.

- When identifying a therapeutic response, the empathetic response usually takes priority.

- When giving information about a procedure, keep in mind the accuracy of the information.

Practice Session: Learning to Answer Implementation Questions

The nurse is caring for a very depressed psychiatric client. When approached by the nurse, the client says, "Don't bother me. I don't have anything worth saying. Go find someone you can help." Which response by the nurse would be most appropriate?

1. "OK. I'll go now and be back in a half hour."
2. "I have the feeling that I upset you. Don't you want to talk to me?"
3. "I'm assigned to take care of you, and I intend to spend time with you."
4. "I would like to stay with you for a while."

Critical Elements	
Key words:	See bold print
Client:	A very depressed psychiatric client
Issue:	Appropriate nursing response to the client's expressions of worthlessness and hopelessness
Type of Stem:	True response stem

Eliminate Options

The nurse is caring for a **very depressed** psychiatric client. When approached by the nurse, the client says, **"Don't bother me. I don't have anything worth saying.** Go find someone you can help." Which response by the nurse would be **most appropriate**?

■ 1. "OK. I'll go now and be back in a half hour."
This NONTHERAPEUTIC *response fails to respond at all to the client's feelings and would be* UNSAFE *because it results in the nurse leaving a very depressed client alone. Depression is caused by feelings of worthlessness and leaving the client reinforces feelings of worthlessness. Monitoring for suicide is necessary and leaving the client alone would be unsafe. Maslow's theory can be used as a guideline here. Maintaining the client's safety is a priority.*

■ 2. "I have the feeling that I upset you. Don't you want to talk to me?"
This response BLOCKS *communication by addressing an inappropriate person (the nurse). The response must be client-centered. Also, the nurse is inappropriately assuming responsibility for the client's feelings. It is not the nurse's fault that the client is feeling this way.*

■ 3. "I'm assigned to take care of you, and I intend to spend time with you." *This authoritarian response BLOCKS communication. The nurse-client relationship is built on trust and collaboration. A response that makes the nurse an authority figure is never therapeutic. The focus of the relationship is to encourage the client's decision-making abilities. This response also fails to address the client's feelings.*

➕ **4. "I would like to stay with you for a while."** *This therapeutic response uses the communication TOOL of offering self. This response conveys to the client a sense of importance and worthiness. It also results in the nurse's staying with the client, which provides for the client's safety. This very depressed client is at risk for suicide.*

A 30-year-old client is admitted to the hospital with chronic renal disease. A two-day-a-week hemodialysis program has just been planned. The client says, "Once in a while I have a pain, but I just ignore it and keep on doing what I have to do." In recognizing that the client's statement indicates denial, what should the nurse do next?

12 DRILL

1. Respond by saying that the client may be avoiding the problem and point out that the client does have certain limitations.
2. Reflect the comment by restating the thought in similar but slightly different words and phrases.
3. Analyze the client's reason for using a defense mechanism and its value at the present time.
4. Follow the client's lead and minimize the importance of the physical limitations imposed by the illness.

Critical Elements	
Key words:	See bold print
Client:	A client with chronic renal disease
Issue:	Denial
Type of Stem:	True response stem

12 ANALYSIS

Eliminate Options

A 30-year-old client was admitted to the hospital with **chronic renal disease.** A two-day-a-week hemodialysis program has just been planned. The client says, "Once in a while I have a pain **but I just ignore it** and keep on doing what I have to do." In **recognizing** that the client's statement indicates **denial,** what should the nurse **do next?**

■ 1. Respond by saying that the client may be avoiding the problem and point out that the client does have certain limitations.
This authoritarian response is NONTHERAPEUTIC. *The nurse is advising the client. Instead, the nurse-client relationship should be collaborative. The nurse needs to help the client resolve the problem by encouraging self-competency. This authoritative approach destroys the client's capabilities to act in self-interest.*

? 2. Reflect the comment by restating the thought in similar but slightly different words and phrases.
This might be a POSSIBILITY; *however, a reflecting comment is used to clarify the meaning of the client's statement. The question asserts that the nurse recognizes the client's statement indicates denial, so an additional clarification statement becomes less attractive.*

➕ **3. Analyze the client's reason for using a defense mechanism and its value at the present time.**
The nurse has already assessed the client's use of denial. What should the nurse DO NEXT? *The* NEXT STEP IN THE NURSING PROCESS *is to* ANALYZE *why the client is using this defense mechanism. This implementation question is a good example of the use of the nursing process in a test question. Note that the test-taking strategy of looking for similar words can also be applied to this question. The idea of "denial" in the stem of the question is repeated in this option by using the words "defense mechanism." This is a very difficult question!*

■ 4. Follow the client's lead and minimize the importance of the physical limitations imposed by the illness.
This INAPPROPRIATE *nursing action would reinforce the client's denial.*

DRILL 13

An upper GI test is ordered for a client. In preparing the client for this test, the nurse should:

1. Withhold all food, drink, and oral medications after 8:00 p.m. on the evening prior to the test.
2. Explain to the client that the prescribed barium preparation will taste chalky.
3. Put the client on a high-residue diet for two or three days prior to the test to cleanse the bowel.
4. Administer morphine as a premedication about one hour prior to the test.

Critical Elements	
Key words:	See bold print
Client:	A client who is to recieve an upper GI
Issue:	Preparing a client for an upper GI
Type of Stem:	True response stem

Eliminate Options

An **upper GI** test is ordered for a client. In **preparing** the client for this test, the nurse **should**:

▬ 1. Withhold all food, drink and oral medications after 8:00 p.m. on the evening prior to the test.
This is INAPPROPRIATE. *The client should receive nothing by mouth from* MIDNIGHT *the night before the exam.*

✚ **2. Explain to the client that the prescribed barium preparation will taste chalky.**
This is the only APPROPRIATE *nursing action. The barium drink that is used to help visualize the upper GI tract is an odorless, tasteless, but has a chalky substance.*

▬ 3. Put the client on a high-residue diet for two or three days prior to the test to cleanse the bowel.
This is INAPPROPRIATE, *since there is no diet restriction prior to this procedure.*

▬ 4. Administer morphine as a premedication about one hour prior to the test.
This is INAPPROPRIATE. *A different premedication drug is given for this procedure.*

EVALUATION

Nursing Behaviors Associated with the Evaluation Phase of the Nursing Process
• Comparing actual outcomes with expected outcomes of therapy
• Determining the impact of nursing actions
• Verifying that tests or measurements were performed correctly
• Evaluating client understanding of information given

When answering questions that focus on the evaluation process, keep in mind the following:

- There may be questions about how the nurse should monitor, or make a judgment concerning, a client's response to therapy or a nursing action.

- Some evaluation questions may have a false response stem. For example, a question may ask about a client's statement that indicates inaccurate information or lack of motivation.

Practice Session: Learning to Answer Evaluation Questions

DRILL 14

A client has a long leg cast on the left leg, applied after sustaining a fracture. Which occurrence would suggest that the nurse should call the physician to determine if bivalving the cast is indicated? The:

1. Client complains of pressure over the area of the left medial malleolus.
2. Client complains of severe itching between the left knee and the left ankle.
3. Client reports pain in the left leg while sitting up in a chair.
4. Nurse assesses poor capillary filling time with tingling in the toes of the left foot.

ANALYSIS 14

Critical Elements	
Key words:	See bold print
Client:	A client with a long leg cast
Issue:	Determining the need to bivalve a cast
Type of Stem:	True response stem

Eliminate Options

A client has a **long leg cast** on the **left** leg applied after sustaining a fracture. Which **occurrence** would suggest that the nurse should **call the physician** to determine if **bivalving the cast** is indicated?

1. The client complains of pressure over the area of the left medial malleolus.
   This is a POSSIBILITY. Complaints of pressure over bony prominences are normal. If the pressure is severe, a window is cut into the cast to alleviate the pressure.

■ 2. The client complains of severe itching between the left knee and the left ankle.
This is a normal manifestation after a cast is applied and does not suggest that the physician needs to be notified.

■ 3. The client reports pain in the left leg while sitting up in a chair.
Pain is expected after a fracture and when a cast is applied, as well as during the healing process. Pain that increases in intensity and duration would need to be assessed.

■ **4. The nurse assesses poor capillary filling time with tingling in the toes of the left foot.**
This is a sign of circulatory constriction and REQUIRES IMMEDIATE ATTENTION *to relieve the constriction. In the evaluation process, the nurse understands that swelling caused by trauma and edema can cause obliteration of blood supply and cause peripheral nerve damage.*

After a myocardial infarction, a client is maintained on a daily dose of digoxin (Lanoxin). The nurse is preparing the client for discharge. Which statement by the client would indicate to the nurse that the client needs further instruction?

1. "I should take my pill every morning at breakfast time."
2. "If I feel nauseated, I will take my antacid and go to bed."
3. "If my pulse goes below 60, I should not take my medicine."
4. "I'll start exercising as soon as my doctor says it is OK."

Critical Elements	
Key words:	See bold print
Client:	A client being discharged after a myocardial infarction
Issue:	Success of pre-discharge teaching
Type of Stem:	False response stem

Eliminate Options

After a **myocardial infarction,** a client is maintained on a daily dose of **digoxin (Lanoxin).** The nurse is preparing the client for **discharge.** Which statement by the client would indicate to the nurse that the client **needs further instruction**?

■ 1. "I should take my pill every morning at breakfast time."
This statement by the client indicates an ACCURATE understanding of how to care for this health problem. Digoxin is usually taken once a day in the morning. This statement would not indicate a need for further instruction.

✚ **2. "If I feel nauseated, I will take my antacid and go to bed."**
This statement indicates an INACCURATE UNDERSTANDING of potential danger signs associated with this medication and a need for further instruction. Nausea can be a manifestation of digitalis toxicity. Instead of going to bed, the client needs to understand that the nausea requires close monitoring and the attention of the physician. Note the "logic" of this question, which has a false response stem.

■ 3. "If my pulse goes below 60, I should not take my medicine."
This statement shows that the client UNDERSTANDS how to monitor for early signs of a toxic effect of digitalis, and what to do if this occurs. Bradycardia, or a pulse rate below 60, may indicate a toxic effect of the drug, and the medicine should be withheld until the doctor is notified. Digitalis toxicity is a life-threatening situation.

■ 4. "I'll start exercising as soon as my doctor says it is OK."
Since this question has a false response stem you can eliminate this statement that indicates an ACCURATE understanding by the client. All cardiac clients should consult with their doctor before placing additional strain on the heart by exercising. The amount of exercise is determined by the degree of damage to the heart muscle. This needs to be assessed by the physician.

Chapter 8

HOW TO TAKE A TIMED NURSING EXAM

Pacing Strategy:
How Can I Be Sure That I Finish in Time?

If you are often among the last students to finish your nursing exams, then the prospect of taking timed exams can be very stressful. Learning to pace yourself during an exam not only will help you finish the exam in the time allowed, but, more importantly, it will improve your score.

NCLEX-RN candidates should recognize that **good pacing skills are essential for the NCLEX-RN.** This is true, even though most candidates report that they found the allotted time to be adequate and about two-thirds of the candidates finish before the time is up. If you are preparing for the NCLEX-RN, practicing your pacing strategy will give you good practice in focusing on test-taking essentials: identifying the critical elements, eliminating incorrect options, and applying test-taking strategies when you are unsure of the answer.

> **Pacing strategy will keep you from becoming stalled and frustrated when you confront very difficult questions, in addition to keeping you focused on the questions and ensuring that you have enough time to complete an exam. Finally, using pacing strategy to improve your concentration and maintain your energy level will help prevent distraction and fatigue.**

"Once over, easy" is a time-saving strategy that you may already know for taking a timed pencil-and-paper exam. "Once over, easy," means that you go through the entire exam the first time answering only those questions that you can answer easily. After you've answered all the "easy" questions, you return to the more difficult ones.

Unfortunately, it is not possible to skip or return to questions on the computerized NCLEX-RN Exam, but this strategy is still worth practicing and using in your course exams.

The strategy of "Once over, easy" is useful because it ensures that you get credit for everything that you are certain you know and about which you can feel confident. In addition, after establishing a pattern of success with the easy questions, you will be better able to correctly answer the difficult questions when you return to them. Often during an exam one question can provide a memory jog that helps you remember information to answer other questions.

When you return to the difficult questions, be sure to use your test-taking strategies. Answer the difficult questions with the confidence that you will be able to correctly answer at least half of them. **Remember that you should not change the answers of questions you previously answered without a very good reason, since your first choice is more likely to be right.**

For NCLEX-RN candidates as well as nursing candidates, the essence of pacing strategy is to plan and monitor how quickly you are answering the questions. This is the best way to ensure that you will be able to answer all the questions in the time allowed.

It is essential to practice using the pacing strategy by answering practice questions in preparation for your exam. Practicing pacing strategy will increase your test-taking speed and accuracy, and will help you fine-tune your ability to use the test-taking techniques and strategies you have learned in *Test Question Logic (TQLogic™) for the NCLEX-RN Exam*. In fact, using pacing strategy while answering practice questions during your review for the NCLEX-RN Exam is one of the best methods of preparing to take the NCLEX-RN.

Steps for the Pacing Strategy

- Immediately after you are allowed to begin, check the time. Make sure your watch is working! If not, use the clock in the room. If you are taking the NCLEX-RN, a "clock" will also be displayed on the screen.

- Determine how many questions there are on the exam, and identify the question that is **ten questions past halfway through the exam.** For example, if there are 80 questions, identify question number 50.

- Depending on how much time you are allowed to take the test, figure out **what time it will be halfway through.** For example, if you are allowed 90 minutes to complete your nursing course exam, calculate what time it will be when you are 45 minutes into the test.

- Begin answering the questions, using your test-taking techniques and your test-taking strategies. On pencil-and-paper exams, skip and do not answer any question:

    a. For which you cannot choose between two choices because they both appear to be right—and you cannot identify a test-taking strategy to help you decide which is best.

    b. That you do not understand.

- Write the question number of each question that you skipped on a piece of paper (e.g., at the top of the paper you are given for your math calculations). These questions then will be easy to locate when returning to them.

- **Try to spend less than one minute per test question. This speed is your goal.** Do not allow any question to immobilize you! Be sure to use your test-taking strategies when you cannot answer a question using your nursing knowledge alone. Make your best selection, and move on to the next question.

- Check the time. When half the time has elapsed, you should be answering the question that is **10 past half way.**

    a. If you are not yet at that question, you'll know that you must work more quickly during the second half of the exam.

    b. If you are already past that question, you may work a bit more slowly during the second half of the exam.

- When you have finished going through the exam the first time, go back and answer the questions you skipped. Remember, when you use your test-taking strategies you have a better than 50/50 chance of answering these questions correctly.

> **When studying for an exam, use pacing strategy every time you answer a set of practice questions. Practice is the only way to increase your speed and accuracy.**

What does it take to ace your nursing course exams—or even to ace the NCLEX-RN Exam on your first try? **Practice, practice, practice!** It is important to emphasize that, as your skill in answering test questions increases, so does your reading speed and comprehension.

When I Finish an Exam, Should I Take Another Look?

Take all the time that you are given! If you find that you finish with time left over, reread the exam. Perhaps you made an error because you misread something in a question. But remember to change an answer **ONLY** if you have misread the information or if other questions helped you to clarify information. Otherwise, it is safest to stick to your first answer.

What Should I Do If I Keep Changing My Answers When Taking an Exam?

One of the most unfortunate—and most common—problems in taking multiple-choice tests is **changing correct answers to incorrect ones.** This causes some students to fail exams.

When answering test questions, always go with your "gut" feeling. This means that you may select an answer for a reason that you are not able to define. You may just like one choice better than another, and it may be difficult to explain why. Trust yourself and choose the answer that you like—and don't change your answer unless you are sure of your reason for doing so! This principle is also true when taking the computerized NCLEX-RN.

Test-taking anxiety and nervousness are two main reasons why students change answers. When you become nervous while answering a difficult question, this anxiety causes you to lose self-confidence. When you lose self-confidence, even if you have some idea about the question, you feel that you cannot trust your own judgment. Then you end up choosing the opposite of your first hunch or "gut" feeling.

You will increase your self-confidence by answering many practice questions. You can also prove to yourself how many times your "gut" feelings are correct by marking questions answered using this strategy during your practice sessions, and computing how many of these questions were answered correctly.

What Should I Do If I Have Trouble Concentrating?

Concentration during any exam is crucial. Your ability to concentrate helps you to notice the key words and select the correct answers.

As you learned in the introduction to *Test Question Logic (TQLogic™) for the NCLEX-RN Exam,* practicing for the test by answering test questions also increases your ability to concentrate. Reviewing in the library, rather than at home, is a good strategy for improving your concentration when answering practice questions—and you will build good concentration habits that way.

If you are nervous and distracted when you are starting an exam, use a relaxation technique and try the first few questions. Students frequently report that after they start answering the first few questions on an exam, they even forget that anyone else is in the room.

As an informed test taker, you should learn to identify signs of poor concentration. Poor concentration can cause you to misread the test question and answer incorrectly. You need to identify those things that prevent you from answering questions correctly. The following table contains a list of common distractions that you may experience when you are losing your concentration.

Common Signs of Distraction

- You feel a sudden physical discomfort such as a neckache or backache
- You get a real craving for food
- You hear noise from another test-taker (e.g., someone chewing gum or tapping a pencil)
- You feel extremely tired
- You read the same question many times over
- You start to think about your vacation

If you notice these signs of distraction occurring during the exam, take a few minutes to breathe deeply, stretch any achy muscles, and then get back on track. Aim for completing just the next few questions without any distractions. Just as it often happens at the beginning of the exam, concentration can quickly be reestablished, and those next few questions can lead seamlessly into the rest of the exam. Refocusing takes just a few seconds. Don't put it off if you find yourself becoming distracted.

Points to Remember

- Pace yourself during the exam.

- After finishing the exam, make use of all the time you have left. Reread the exam.

- Never change answers unless you misread a part of the question or if other questions helped you to clarify information.

- Be confident! You now have the nursing knowledge and the test-taking skills to succeed.

Chapter 9

HOW TO PREPARE FOR THE NCLEX-RN EXAM

Your Personalized Review Program

The time has come to review all of the nursing content you have learned up until now! To help you gain control, this chapter will help you organize a personalized review program.

An important consideration in tailoring your personal study program is identifying your study needs and focusing on your specific weak areas. The information provided in this chapter may be exactly what is needed by the average student. However, some students may need more preparation in some areas and less in others. Your review plan and your study schedule will depend upon your own specific needs and your identification of your own weak areas.

Plan to spend one-third of your study time reviewing nursing content and two-thirds of your study time answering test questions.

The following seven-step program is a recommended guidelines for preparing to ace the NCLEX-RN:

Seven-Step Study Program

1. Orientation—Identify the Structure of the NCLEX-RN
2. Prepare to Invest the Time It Takes
3. Plan Your Comprehensive Review
4. Choose Your Materials
5. Complete at least 3,000 Questions Before the Exam
6. Review the Steps to Studying
7. Assess Your Progress

You have already made a significant investment in yourself by successfully completing your nursing program. You have demonstrated the ability to be committed, dedicated, determined, and motivated. Your next goal is to become licensed. Once you set your mind on this goal, it will be easier for you to follow through with your study program.

STEP 1 | ORIENTATION: IDENTIFY THE STRUCTURE OF THE NCLEX-RN

Remember—your goal now is simply to pass the NCLEX-RN. Therefore, when you plan your review, you should be careful to include only the essential information needed to pass the NCLEX-RN.

Although the NCLEX-RN covers all clinical areas, the exam does not test everything you learned in nursing school! The purpose of the NCLEX-RN is actually rather limited: it is designed to demonstrate whether you are capable of practicing safely and effectively at the beginning level of professional nursing. Therefore, your review should focus on what will be on the exam; don't waste precious review time studying inessential material.

The NCLEX-RN test plan is your official guide to what will be covered. Most beginning nurses practice in the acute care setting, and they deal with clients with acute medical/surgical disorders. This knowledge is what is emphasized on the NCLEX-RN. The NCLEX-RN structure emphasizes key nursing concepts and is organized according to two major components: the nursing process and client needs . Take a moment now to review the concepts outlined in following tables.

The NCLEX-RN Test Plan

Five Categories of the Nursing Process

(1) Assessment	17-23%*
(2) Analysis	17-23%
(3) Planning	17-23%
(4) Implementation	17-23%
(5) Evaluation	17-23%

Four Categories of Client Needs

Safe, Effective Care Environment
1. Management of care   13-19%*
2. Safety and Infection control   8-14%*

Health Promotion and Maintenance   6-12%*

Psychosocial Integrity   6-12%*

Physiological Integrity
1. Basic care and comfort   6-12%*
2. Pharmacological and parenteral therapies   13-19%*
3. Reduction of risk potential   13-19%*
4. Physiological adaptation   11-17%*

* Refers to the combined percentage of test questions in each category.

Integrated Concepts and Processes

- Nursing Process
- Caring
- Communication and Documentation
- Teaching/Learning

NOTE: Content distribution for the NCLEX-RN according to the Test Plan for the National Council Licensure Examination for Registered Nurses.

How to Review Nursing Content

To plan your review of essential nursing knowledge for the NCLEX-RN, it is helpful to organize the material into the four major clinical areas: medical/surgical, psychiatric, pediatrics, and maternal/child nursing.

Then, for a comprehensive review in the medical/surgical and pediatrics clinical settings, use a body-systems approach and group the disorders according to the related body system.

Sequence of Nursing Content for Review

1. Review the medical/surgical disorders.
- Spend the greatest amount of time reviewing medical/surgical content. Note that 50% of the questions focus on this area.
- Use the body-systems approach.
- Begin by understanding pathophysiology.
- Identify early manifestations of life-threatening complications.
- Include drugs associated with each disease and highlight early signs of toxicity.
- Review problems of the aged client with acute medical/surgical conditions.

2. Review the psychiatric disorders.
- Clarify these disorders, since they cause the greatest amount of confusion.
- Clarify major nursing intervention for behaviors associated with each disorder.
- Identify the drugs associated with each disorder and differentiate between side and toxic effects.
- Identify therapeutic communication techniques. (Note that this is a thread identified in all four categories of clients needs.)
- Review how to communicate with the confused and aging client.

3. Briefly review maternal/child nursing.
- Concentrate on high-risk pregnancy. Review the gynecological procedures, such as hysterectomy or radium insertion for cancer of the cervix.
- Identify the drugs associated with each condition and differentiate between side and toxic effects.

4. Review the pediatric conditions.
- Use a body-systems approach as it relates to pediatrics.
- Include growth and development, especially of infants, toddlers and preschoolers.
- Identify the drugs associated with each condition and differentiate between side and toxic effects.
- Identify appropriate play materials at each stage of growth.
- Review acute pediatric conditions in a hospital setting.

5. Review these special areas:
- Review basic management.
- Practice math calculations, especially drip rates.
- Identify therapeutic diets associated with each disorder and foods included in and excluded from therapeutic diets.
- Review basic safety measures, such as transferring a client from a bed to a wheelchair or cart, administering medications, and walking with a blind client.

PREPARE TO INVEST THE TIME IT TAKES

And it does take time! You will need to set aside the time that is necessary to review the nursing content, and the time it will take to improve your skill in answering test questions.

Perhaps you think that you will not be able to spend much time studying because of all your other obligations and commitments. At this time, it is critical to remember that your goal is to become a licensed professional registered nurse. You may need to arrange to take time off from work or hire a babysitter to achieve your goal. If possible, you also need to put your family or personal problems "on hold" until after the exam. Your priority at this time is to prepare to pass the NCLEX-RN Exam on your first try.

Your 30-Day Schedule

You can prepare comprehensively and efficiently for the NCLEX-RN if you plan your review carefully. A basic one-month time schedule that covers the essential information is detailed below. Use your common sense to modify the time schedule to meet your individual studying needs. If you feel you have no special considerations, follow the plan exactly as shown.

Suggested Time Schedule	
Clinical settings:	
Medical-Surgical & Pharmacology	14 days
Psychiatric & Pharmacology	6 days
Pediatric & Pharmacology	3 days
Maternal-Child & Pharmacology	3 days
Management & Pharmacology	2 days
Other areas*	2 days
Total Time:	30 days
* A minimum of two days is planned to cover math calculations, nutrition, growth and development, and any areas that you find particularly difficult.	

Use the two last days to review any remaining areas of weakness and take additional practice tests. Be sure to leave these two days clear when you make your four-week review plan.

After reviewing Step 3, you will have a better idea of any special modifications you may need to make to ensure that your review plan and time schedule better suits your needs. Use the 30-Day Study Calendar on page 111 to plot your personal study plan. In designing your personal comprehensive study program, it is necessary to develop both a daily and a weekly schedule. Set up your schedule now—or it will soon be too late to complete a thorough review.

Your Detailed Daily Personal Study Plan

- **Clinical setting:** Define the clinical focus.

- **Body system:** Begin with the system that is the most difficult.

- **Review book:** Purchase a content review book and identify the sections to be covered. Keep a nursing manual handy for reference, but only use textbooks when needed to clarify a problem area.

- **Tests:** Review at least 3,000 questions using the strategies outlined in this book.

Now you will have an idea of the specific nursing content you will cover on a daily basis, the amount of time required to invest in studying, the resources you will use, and the kinds and numbers of questions you must answer. Use the 30-Day Study Calendar to custom design your personal study program.

Set a personal goal for each day of the four weeks prior to taking the NCLEX-RN. Specify the area to be reviewed and the questions to be answered during your planned study periods. Make sure each body system and every clinical setting is covered.

PLAN YOUR COMPREHENSIVE REVIEW

As mentioned earlier, when reviewing essential nursing knowledge, it is helpful to organize the material into the four major clinical settings: medical/surgical, psychiatric, pediatrics, and maternal/child nursing. There are some other special areas to be covered as well. For each disorder, the nursing content that should be reviewed is detailed in the table on the following page.

Guidelines for Studying a Disorder

1. **Define the disorder** in the basic terms of the pathophysiological processes that occur.

2. Identify and distinguish between **early** and **late manifestations** of the disorder and the related nursing interventions.

3. Identify the most important and **life-threatening** complications. (Remember, you are safest when you can assess early characteristics of life-threatening complications.)

4. Determine the **medical treatment** for the disorder. Note the nursing interventions.

5. Identify the **teaching-learning** needs associated with prevention of, or adaptation to, the disorder. This includes skills, information, or other help needed to cope.

When you plan your review of nursing information content in the medical/surgical clinical setting, identify the body system where your knowledge is weakest.

Begin by studying your most difficult body system first. Then, be sure to use the guidelines in previous table to study each body system and its associated disorders.

CHOOSE YOUR REVIEW BOOK AND/OR RESOURCE MATERIAL

Clearly, you will need reference materials specifically designed to help you study for the NCLEX-RN. **Class notes are too extensive;** they contain material that helped you pass your nursing program exams, but which may not be essential for the NCLEX-RN. Your textbooks are also too extensive and reviewing them all would be overwhelming!

This is why MEDS provides the *NCLEX-RN Exam Essentials Review* book in outline form. Be sure to use a book such as this to study the nursing content. Refer to a textbook only when you need to further clarify information.

MEDS also provides this review on CD-ROM.

ANSWER AT LEAST 3,000 TEST QUESTIONS

Answering practice test questions that simulate those found on the NCLEX-RN exam will help you master the skill of learning to read and interpret multiple choice questions correctly. Frequent practice test-taking sessions offer you the opportunity to perfect your pacing technique and become comfortable using test-taking strategies. Practice questions also enable you to apply your knowledge and give you the opportunity to instantly assess what you have learned. When you answer practice questions, you are:

- Clarifying nursing information

- Developing your safety judgment

- Integrating key concepts such as nursing process, communication, documentation, accountability, and growth and development

- Polishing your analytical thinking skills

One myth about preparing for the NCLEX-RN exam is that "the more you memorize, the better prepared you will be." Since the exam focuses on your ability to make safe judgments as a beginning nurse, memorizing facts is only a small part of the preparation process. Most students have the greatest difficulty in applying the nursing information to the practice of nursing. Q&A practice is absolutely essential in preparing for the NCLEX-RN!*

Review the Steps to Studying

1. Did I begin by using a body-systems approach?

2. Did I pay special attention to the medical-surgical clinical setting?

3. Did I identify the system that is my greatest weakness? (Look at the major sections and subsections, and assess your strengths and weaknesses. Emphasize your problem areas in your review plan.)

4. Did I review the weak areas that I identified in Step 3?

5. Does my study plan include answering a minimum of 3,000 test questions (about 100 questions a day)

7 STEP

ASSESS YOUR PROGRESS

Once you have begun your personal study program and started answering practice test questions, be sure to use the assessment scale provided in Table 7 to help you navigate the direction of your study plan. By using the scale, you will systematically move from the areas you have mastered to the areas where you are weakest, until you have covered all areas necessary to build the skills needed to pass the NCLEX-RN.

Each time you answer a set of questions, calculate and record the percentage of questions that you answered correctly. To assess your progress in each questions type, use the following chart.

Assessment Scale for Practice Tests

Score	Recommendation
95% +	**Superior!** Don't spend additional time on this area. Feel very confident.
85-94%	**Very Good.** Only return to this area after you have remedied all deficiencies. Feel confident.
74-84%	**Average.** Success in this area is questionable. Repeat until score is above 75%. Keep answering questions and work on building confidence. You might wish to briefly review the methods outlined in this book to make sure you are interpreting the questions correctly.
Below 75%	**Warning Signal!** Spend lots of time reviewing this area and don't cut corners! If you feel that your understanding of nursing content is adequate, be sure to review your test-taking skills, and then retest this area using all of the applicable strategies.

Be sure to complete your outline and draft your calendar so you know you have time to finish your program before taking the NCLEX-RN exam. If you follow the steps we have outlined for you, you will build the skills and the confidence you need to pass on your first try.

Last but not least, you need to learn about the computerized NCLEX-RN format and plan to spend some time using your home computer or your learning lab.

How Does "Computerized Adaptive Testing" Work?

The NCLEX-RN exam is now computerized and is officially called the NCLEX/CAT-RN Exam. "CAT" stands for "Computerized Adaptive Testing." The computerized exam "adapts" the exam to the skill level of each individual candidate who takes the test.

The computer contains a "bank" of about 3,000 test questions. When the candidate begins to answer the questions, the computer uses the selected answers to measure the candidate's level of ability and then selects the next question at that candidate's level of ability. This process continues throughout the exam.

Adaptive testing is based upon the testing principle that questions that are too difficult or too easy for a given candidate do not measure that candidate's knowledge as accurately as questions more suited to that candidate's ability. The testing continues until a pattern of responses demonstrating a passing (or failing) level of competence is established.

Is This Fair?

Adaptive testing is fair because **the test plan for the computerized NCLEX-RN exam is the same for all candidates, and all candidates must still demonstrate the same level of nursing competence** in order to pass the exam. As the candidate continues to answer questions, the computer selects questions in all four areas of client needs, using all five phases of the nursing process.

With adaptive testing, candidates with high ability who correctly answer questions at a higher level—questions which are more difficult—will not have to answer questions at a lower level. Such candidates can demonstrate their ability to apply their nursing knowledge by answering a smaller number of high-level questions. On the other hand, candidates with more average abilities are given the same opportunity to demonstrate their competence by answering a larger number of questions at a less advanced level.

The National Council of Nursing has done extensive national testing of the NCLEX/CAT-RN Exam, and has found that it fairly and accurately measures the ability and nursing knowledge of all candidates

What Computer Skills Do I Need?

You will not need any special computer skills to take the NCLEX-RN.

The exam uses a special color-coded keyboard. To select your answers, you need to use the mouse to move the cursor on the screen to the desired location.

Is There Any Way to Practice Using the NCLEX-RN Computer Format?

Although you do not actually need computer skills to take the NCLEX-RN Exam, you will be more comfortable and more confident when taking the exam if you first practice taking some computerized exams using the same format.

The CD provided with *Test Question Logic (TQLogic™) for the NCLEX-RN Exam* includes the same questions that are found in Chapter Ten—the Final Exam, but in NCLEX format. The CD also includes complete rationales for all correct and incorrect answers, and a special Personalized Performance Analysis feature to assess your progress. For additional support, try MEDS' StarNurse Exam-A-Day Gold Online. It can be purchased at www.medspub.com.

What Do the Questions on the NCLEX-RN Exam Look Like?

On your computer screen, you will see a special format that includes separate boxes that contain the **case scenario**, the **stem** of the test question, and the **four options**. The screen will look like this:

In preparing to administer a medication to a confused elderly client, the nurse discovers that the client does not have an identification bracelet on. The client states that the medication has already been taken. Which of the following nursing actions provides for the client's safety?

☐   1. Ask if the client might be confused about taking the medication.

Case Scenario and Stem

☐   2. Identify the client based upon which bed is occupied in the room.

☐   3. Check the client's chart and ask another health care worker to identify the client.

☐   4. Ask the client's name and then obtain an identification bracelet for the client.

Four Options

When you use the color-coded keys to highlight, select and enter your answer, the computer records your answer and selects the next question at your ability level. Then the next question appears on the screen.

How is the Exam Scored?

The NCLEX-RN Exam is scored according to a weighted formula that takes into account the number of questions answered correctly and the difficulty levels of the questions. There is no extra penalty for wrong answers, but it is not possible to skip questions on the computerized exam.

How is the Exam Timed?

The maximum amount of time allowed is five hours, with a ten-minute break after the second hour. Only about one-third of the candidates require the entire five hours to complete the exam. A running "clock" will appear on the computer screen, so it will be easy for you to keep track of time.

With the new computerized technology, the test can be given year-round and in more convenient locations—and the test results can be sent to the State Boards of Nursing within 48 hours!

Since the Test Adapts to My Skill Level, Why Do I Need to Use Test-Taking Strategies?

You need good test-taking skills to make the most of your nursing knowledge on the NCLEX-RN and achieve a passing score. The test-taking techniques and strategies you will learn in the MEDS' *Test Question Logic (TQLogic™) for the NCLEX-RN Exam* book will help you understand the questions better and will keep you focused on what each question is asking.

In addition, because it is not possible to skip questions on the computerized NCLEX-RN, it is very important for you to know some test-taking strategies you can use when you are unsure of the answer. When taking a computerized exam, it is important not to become upset if a question is too difficult. Your test-taking strategies will give you some guidelines to follow on difficult questions so that you can improve your chances of selecting the best option and then go right on to the next question. Pacing yourself is important, too, to ensure you will have enough time to complete the exam.

COMPUTERIZED NCLEX-RN EXAM

EXAM SETTING:
Administered in small rooms that allow for privacy and quiet during the exam. Sites accommodate up to 25 candidates at once.

EQUIPMENT:
The special NCLEX/CAT-RN computer, with two special color-coded keys to select and enter answers. No computer skills are needed. However, you should practice answering sample computerized questions before taking the exam, in order to become comfortable with this format. A small "clock" is displayed on the screen.

Scratch paper is provided for calculations.

MATERIAL COVERED:
Covers entire range of nursing content, from all clinical areas.

TYPES OF QUESTIONS AND TEST PLAN:
Consists of multiple choice test questions with four options and only one correct answer and Alternate Test Item Formats.

Uses the four categories of client needs and the five phases of the nursing process.

Consists only of independent test questions. Most questions include a brief description of a clinical situation, but each question stands alone and is not linked to other questions.

NUMBER OF QUESTIONS ASKED AND TIME ALLOWED:
Each candidate answers questions selected according to his or her own level of ability. No two candidates will take the same exam, but all must demonstrate the same level of competence.

Each candidate must answer between 75 and 265 questions in five hours.

TEST-TAKING STRATEGIES:
There is no penalty for incorrect answers—and you CANNOT skip questions.

Use a test-taking strategy if you can't decide between the two best options, don't know the answer, or don't understand the question. Test-taking strategies are essential to maximize your score—and to prevent becoming stalled or upset when answering difficult questions.

PACING:

Do not spend too long on any one question.

You MUST answer each question, in sequence, and you cannot return to previous questions. However, the questions are selected according to your level of skill.

REQUIREMENT FOR PASSING:

The NCLEX-RN candidate must demonstrate knowledge above the minimum passing standard by:

1. Correctly answering a minimum of 75 test questions at a high level of difficulty; or

2. Answering 75 to 265 test questions with a final weighted competence measure above the passing standard; or

3. Achieving a competence measure above the passing standard for the last 60 questions answered.

CHANGING ANSWERS AND REVIEWING QUESTIONS:

Answers are "selected" with the mouse and can only be deselected BEFORE you press the NEXT key. Once you enter your answer to a question, you cannot change it.

At the end of the exam, you cannot review the test questions.

HOW TO PREPARE FOR THE EXAM:

The NCLEX-RN encompasses all clinical areas, so you need to plan a comprehensive review.

Use the *Test Question Logic (TQLogic™) for the NCLEX-RN Exam* book, keeping a nursing manual at hand for reference.

Sharpen your test-taking skills, and answer at least 3,000 practice test questions before the NCLEX-RN Exam.

How to Take the Computerized NCLEX-RN Exam:

1. **Prepare comprehensively** and be sure to be well rested. This is a vital exam!

2. **Read each question carefully,** identifying the **critical elements** in the question as explained in this book.

3. Remember that **each question must be answered in sequence.** You may not skip questions or go back to change your answer once it has been entered.

4. **Use your scratch paper wisely.** Sometimes information from one question may prove helpful in answering a subsequent question. Since it is not possible to return to earlier questions, you may wish to use the scratch paper that is provided for calculations to jot down facts provided in one question which you think you may need in later questions but have trouble recalling.

5. **Don't panic if someone finishes before you!** The test adapts to each candidate's level of ability. This means that you may take longer to prove that you are capable of practicing competently at the beginning level of nursing.

6. **Don't panic if the computer stops after a short time!** This does not mean you failed. The computer stops when the exam is able to determine with at least 95% certainty whether you have demonstrated the ability to practice safely at the minimal level of nursing competence. It is helpful to know that: (1) Approximately one candidate in three will be stopped after about 75 test questions, and more than 50% of those stopped will pass; (2) about 1/3 of the candidates will complete the maximum number of 265 test questions, and about 50% will pass; and (3) approximately 1/3 of the students will fall in the middle of these groups, and about 50% of them will pass.

7. **Keep a positive attitude!** Remember that you have learned a great amount of nursing knowledge, and that the exam is only designed to determine whether you are able to practice safely and effectively at the entry level.

ATTENTION, ALL NCLEX-RN CANDIDATES!

The best approach to building confidence for the NCLEX-RN and decreasing your anxiety is to get as much experience as possible in taking a computer exam.

30-Day Study Calendar

		MED/SURG M/S Endocrine	MED/SURG Oncology/ Immun. Burns	WOMEN'S HEALTH Maternity	MGMT
Sunday		MED/SURG M/S Endocrine	MED/SURG Oncology/ Immun. Burns	WOMEN'S HEALTH Maternity	MGMT
Monday	MED/SURG M/S Fluid	MED/SURG M/S Blood	PSYCHIATRIC Psy Anxiety	Maternity	MGMT PHARM
Tuesday	MED/SURG M/S Resp	PHARM M/S Cardio.	PSYCHIATRIC Psy Schizophrenia	WOMEN'S HEALTH Maternity	
Wednesday	MED/SURG M/S Surgical	PHARM M/S Cardio.	PSYCHIATRIC Psy Mood	PEDIATRICS	
Thursday	MED/SURG M/S GI	MED/SURG M/S Genitourinary	PSYCHIATRIC Psy Chemical/ Pharm	PEDIATRICS PEDS	
Friday	MED/SURG M/S GI	MED/SURG M/S Genitourinary	PSYCHIATRIC Psy Organic Mental Disorders	PEDIATRICS PEDS	
Saturday	MED/SURG M/S Musculoskeletal	MED/SURG M/S Neurologic	PSYCHIATRIC Psy Eating Disorders	MGMT PHARM	

NOTES

Chapter 10

A FINAL EXAM

Be confident and good luck!

Are you ready for the Final Exam?

> **You have your choice of using this chapter or answering the same questions in computerized format using the computer disk enclosed with this book.**

The CD-ROM features the computerized NCLEX-RN screen design, as well as MEDS unique Personal Performance Analysis to automatically assess your performance. The Personal Performance Analysis classifies your answers to the questions according to clinical area and phase of the nursing process. The analysis also calculates your score according to the critical elements in the question, applicable test-taking strategy, and type of question (prioritizing, nursing process, communication, etc.). If you do not have a home computer that uses this type of disk, you may wish to use your nursing program's learning lab.

Students who use this chapter in the book for the Final Exam instead of the disk, should be sure to schedule some practice time on a computer before taking the NCLEX-RN, to become familiar with the computerized format. To use the exam in this chapter, have a pencil ready to record your answers and a piece of paper. You will also need a wristwatch so that you can pace yourself. (The computerized exam displays the time on the screen.)

For a brief review of *Test Question Logic (TQLogic) for the NCLEX-RN Exam,* see the "Points to Remember" at the end of each chapter.

To achieve your best score, take this exam when you are well rested. A relaxed, positive attitude helps. Make sure that you haven't skipped a meal. And make sure that you have a comfortable chair.

Tips for the Final Exam:

- Read each question carefully. If you are taking the exam on paper, circle or underline important words.

- Be sure to identify all four of the critical elements.

- Remember that only one answer in each question is correct, and you receive credit only for correct answers. Of the four options offered with each question, you are looking for the **best** one.

- When you know the type of stem and the issue in the question, make a decision about each option as you read it by using the selection procedure. Be sure you have correctly identified the client in a communication question.

- If you cannot decide which option is the best, use a test-taking strategy; if no strategy seems to apply, follow your gut feeling—and if you don't know, guess! Most exams have no penalty for wrong answers.

- If you are taking the exam on paper, **be sure to record all your answers!** You may also wish to indicate which questions you answered by means of a strategy.

- Pace yourself! This exam has 100 questions, so you should allow yourself approximately **one hour and 40 minutes** to answer the questions. Find the question that is halfway-plus-ten (**Question 60**), and try to finish this question at the end of **50 minutes**. Use your test-taking strategies and use your time wisely!

- If you are preparing for **nursing course exams**, answer the easy questions first and then go back to the difficult ones.

- **Attention, NCLEX-RN candidates:** Do not leave any questions blank! Remember, it is not possible to skip questions or return to previous questions on the computerized NCLEX-RN Exam.

- Concentrate during the exam and be sure to use relaxation techniques as needed.

Good luck! Remember: BONUS test-taking tips and strategies can be found on the enclosed *Test Smart* CD-ROM!

1. A nurse visits a client at home one week following discharge after a myocardial infarction. The client is taking chlorothiazide (Diuril) 500 mg daily and digoxin (Lanoxin) 0.25 mg daily. The nurse should give top priority to assessing the client's knowledge of:

    1. Sources of potassium.
    2. Sources of sodium.
    3. Activity restrictions.
    4. Signs of a heart attack.

2. An adolescent client is to have a water system heating device (K-Pad) applied to a pulled muscle. The client tells the nurse that the device does not feel very warm. The most appropriate nursing action is to:

    1. Explain to the client that these heating devices never feel hot.
    2. Check the temperature setting on the heating unit and feel the pad for warmth.
    3. Call the appropriate repair department and have them fix the unit.
    4. Turn the temperature up on the unit if it doesn't feel warm enough to the client.

3. A client who weighs 288 pounds says to the nurse, "I'm going to have surgery to have my stomach stapled so I can lose weight. I've tried everything else, and nothing seems to work." Which response by the nurse would be therapeutic?

    1. "That's a pretty drastic measure. Are you sure that is what you want to do?"
    2. "I hear that the surgery is only a temporary measure, and if you have the staples removed, you will only gain the weight back again."
    3. "It must be difficult to be overweight and not able to lose weight. What does your spouse think about the surgery?"
    4. "Can you tell me about the possible consequences and side effects of this type of surgery?"

4. The nurse finds an elderly client standing in a puddle of water in the unit's hallway. The nurse does not know this client. What should the nurse do first?

    1. Ask the client's name and room number.
    2. Wipe up the water until the floor is completely dry.
    3. Call the supervisor for assistance in identifying the client.
    4. Have the client wait in the lounge until security arrives.

5. The nurse caring for a client on the evening before a scheduled left below-the-knee amputation provides preoperative teaching, including deep breathing and coughing. Which question would be most helpful for the nurse to ask the client to evaluate the effectiveness of the preoperative teaching?

    1. "Do you understand what we have just discussed about deep breathing and coughing?"
    2. "Do you think that you will need to have a sedative to help you sleep tonight?"
    3. "Will you demonstrate for me the correct method of deep breathing and coughing?"
    4. "Do you have any questions concerning your scheduled surgical procedure?"

6. The nurse is conducting a preoperative interview three days prior to admitting a seven-year-old client for a tonsillectomy. The client's parent requests information to prepare the child for hospitalization. The nurse knows that the child was hospitalized last year for a fractured femur. Which nursing actions would best meet this child's needs for preparation?

    1. Suggest a role play and provide materials.
    2. Remind the child of the experience of the past hospitalization.
    3. Read the child a story about another child having a similar operation.
    4. Tell the child the appointment is only to have the throat checked.

7. A client is admitted to the hospital in respiratory distress. The doctor orders oxygen via mask and the client to be placed in Fowler's position. Which nursing action is most important for this client at this time?

    1. Support and align the hands with the forearms.
    2. Use handrolls.
    3. Raise the head of the bed to allow for greater lung expansion.
    4. Support the feet at right angles to the lower legs.

8. A 23-year-old gravida 1, para 0 is admitted to the hospital at 38 weeks gestation with pregnancy induced hypertension (PIH). Which finding would the nurse identify as inconsistent with the admitting diagnosis?

    1. 3+ protein in the urine.
    2. Deep tendon reflexes of +1.
    3. Blood pressure of 148/98.
    4. 1+ pitting sacral edema.

9. When the nurse enters a client's room, the client's son tells the nurse, "You people can't do anything right. Ever since my parent was admitted to this hospital, it has been one mistake after another. I am taking my parent out of here before you kill my parent." The nurse's most helpful response to the son is:

    1. "You feel that your parent is not being well cared for?"
    2. "We have the best intentions for the clients."
    3. "I'll get the supervisor for you."
    4. "Your parent hasn't complained about the care. What specifically is the problem?"

10. **After a myocardial infarction, which vital signs assessment should the nurse recognize as possible indications of cardiogenic shock?**

    1. BP - 180/100, P - 90, irregular.
    2. BP - 130/80, P - 100 regular.
    3. BP - 90/50, P - 50 regular.
    4. BP - 80/60, P - 110, irregular.

11. **An 18-year-old client is hospitalized for treatment of severe depression. Which nursing approach would be most therapeutic to include in the client's plan of care?**

    1. Giving the client choices.
    2. Spending time with the client.
    3. Providing a chess game.
    4. Encouraging decision-making.

12. **A two-year-old is hospitalized with bacterial pneumonia. The nurse will monitor the client's respiratory status closely. Which manifestations would the nurse identify as the earliest indication of respiratory difficulty?**

    1. Respiratory rate of 40 to 48.
    2. Blood pressure of 80/60.
    3. Cyanosis of mucous membranes.
    4. Circumoral/periorbital pallor.

13. **A client is in labor and is admitted with a blood pressure of 86/52. She is four centimeters dilated and uncomfortable. The nurse should give immediate consideration to which nursing action?**

    1. Call the physician to report the blood pressure.
    2. Turn the client on her side and retake her blood pressure.
    3. Reassure the client that everything is all right.
    4. Ask the client if she would like some pain medication.

14. **During a client's postoperative recovery from an ileostomy, the nurse begins teaching stoma care. The client refuses to look at the ostomy and tells the nurse, "I'd rather be dead than have to live with this all my life." The appropriate nursing response is:**

    1. "I can't imagine what you must be feeling; it must be awful."
    2. "I'll call your physician and see if something can be ordered to help you relax."
    3. "There's no reason to feel like that. Things will get better."
    4. "You appear upset. Would you like to talk?"

15. **A female client was hospitalized for major depression and treated with nortriptyline (Pamelor). As the client is preparing for discharge, which statement by the client would indicate to the nurse the need for further instruction?**

    1. "I'm glad this medicine helps me. My husband and I would like to start our family as soon as possible."
    2. "If I should feel hopeless and suicidal again, I have the telephone number of my therapist to call for help."
    3. "I hope I will not have to continue taking medicine forever. I guess I'll have to see how I do."
    4. "I plan to see my psychiatrist regularly. If I continue to do well, I can probably stop taking my medication in nine to 12 months."

16. **A client who had foot surgery has just returned from the recovery room. The nurse's initial assessment indicates the client is stable. An hour later, the client's roommate turns on the call light and tells the nurse that the client has gotten up and hopped on one foot to the bathroom, using the IV pole for support. The initial nursing action to provide for the client's safety is to:**

    1. Open the bathroom door to assess if the client is okay.
    2. Assist the client in ambulating back to bed and get the client a bedpan.
    3. Explain to the client that it is not safe to be hopping around on one foot.
    4. Get a wheelchair and help the client back to bed when the client is done in the bathroom.

17. **An elderly client was hospitalized for observation after experiencing a fall when walking for exercise. The client is to ambulate for the first time since the fall, but tells the nurse, "I'm afraid to get up." The best response by the nurse is:**

    1. "There is nothing to be afraid of. The order wouldn't have been written if your doctor didn't think that you were ready."
    2. "Tell me what concerns you about getting up today."
    3. "I will have another person here to help you when you get up."
    4. "Are you afraid of falling again?"

18. **To safely assess for correct placement of a nasogastric tube, the nurse should:**

    1. Instill 30 mL of saline to assess client tolerance.
    2. Instill 10 mL of air into the tube and listen for gurgling sounds with a stethoscope over the gastric area.
    3. Aspirate stomach contents with a syringe.
    4. Place the end of the tube in water to assess for bubbling.

19. **A psychiatric client is re-hospitalized after deciding to discontinue prescribed medication. The client has responded well to the support of the nurse-client relationship. The client's discharge plans include living with the parents and attending a job training program during the day. What is the most important goal for the client's remaining sessions with the nurse?**

1. Reinforce the importance of taking the medications as prescribed.
2. Anticipate future problems and how the client might handle them.
3. Terminate the nurse-client relationship.
4. Promote the client's self-confidence.

20. **The nurse knows the discharge teaching for a client with Hepatitis A virus is successful when the client indicates it would be inappropriate to:**

    1. Donate blood.
    2. Eat fried foods.
    3. Vacation in a foreign country.
    4. Order a salad in a restaurant.

21. **A client is hospitalized following myocardial infarction. When transferring the client from a cart to the bed, the priority nursing action is to:**

    1. Ask the client to place the arms on the chest.
    2. Lock the wheels on the cart and the bed.
    3. Have at least four people help with the transfer.
    4. Use a draw sheet to move the client.

22. **The nurse understands the inaccurate statement about reality testing is that it is:**

    1. An ego function.
    2. Impaired in psychotic individuals.
    3. Impaired in persons who are mentally retarded.
    4. The capacity to distinguish thoughts, feelings, fantasies, and other experiences that originate inside the individual from those that are part of the outside environment.

23. **The client is to receive a medication for control of tachycardia and an irregular heart rate. The nurse obtains the following vital signs prior to administering this medication: blood pressure 98/54, pulse 48 bpm., respirations 30, and temperature 98 degrees F. The client's skin is cool, with cyanosis of the fingers and lips. The appropriate nursing action is to:**

    1. Administer the medication as ordered by the physician.
    2. Omit the medication for a day or two, depending on the client's response and manifestations.
    3. Notify the physician concerning the client's status before administering the medication.
    4. Give the client one half of the ordered dose.

24. **The nurse is preparing a teaching plan for a client being discharged following major abdominal surgery. The client will be doing personal dressing changes at home. Which technique is the most important for the nurse to include in the discharge teaching plan?**

    1. Opening bandages properly to maintain their sterility.
    2. Maintaining strict aseptic technique.
    3. Proper gloving technique.
    4. Good handwashing technique.

25. **A premature infant weighed only three pounds and seven ounces at birth. Following a lengthy stay in the hospital, the infant's weight has increased to five pounds so the infant will be discharged soon. Which statement by the mother would indicate to the nurse that additional teaching is needed?**

    1. "My baby is so fragile that I will need to be extra careful with everything I do for the baby."
    2. "I know that my baby will need to see the doctor regularly for awhile, and I have the appointments on my calendar."
    3. "My mother is going to stay with me for several weeks to help me with my older children."
    4. "I have the nursery, clothing, bottles, and diapers all ready for the day we bring our baby home."

26. **The doctor finds a lump in the client's breast and says that a biopsy needs to be done. The client asks the nurse, "Do you think it is cancer?" The initial nursing response should be:**

    1. "You seem to be worried about what the doctor may find."
    2. "Do you have a family history of breast cancer?"
    3. "We won't know anything until the biopsy is done."
    4. "Most lumps are not cancerous, so you really shouldn't worry."

27. **A client has just been diagnosed with advanced, untreatable cancer. When the nurse enters the room to set up the bath equipment, the client says, "I'm not an invalid, you know. I can take care of myself. Get out and leave me alone." What is the best nursing response?**

    1. "I know that you are not an invalid. I was just trying to help you."
    2. "It sounds to me like you are angry about something. Did somebody do something wrong?"
    3. "You are pretty upset. Let's talk about it."
    4. "I'll just set up this equipment for you to bathe and come back later when you're not so angry."

28. **A six-year-old child is admitted with a spiral fracture of the humerus and multiple bruises of the forearm. The physician states that the injuries and other signs are suspicious for abuse. The nurse's initial goal is to:**

    1. Prevent further abuse of the client.
    2. Encourage the client to express any feelings.
    3. Determine who is responsible for the abuse.
    4. Teach the parents the appropriate methods of discipline.

29. **While caring for a client, the nurse should practice good body mechanics to reduce the chance of muscle strain. In using good body mechanics, the nurse would avoid:**

    1. Moving muscles quickly, using short tugs.
    2. Using the longest and strongest muscles of the body.
    3. Leaning toward objects being pushed.
    4. Carrying objects close to the body .

30. An elderly client is admitted to the hospital with pneumonia. The client's daughter, who takes care of the client at home, tells the nurse, "I'm so glad my parent is here. You can provide much better care than I can." The best nursing response to the daughter is:

    1. "We do have the equipment and people to take care of sick clients."
    2. "It is not easy to care for the elderly. How do you manage?"
    3. "Your daughter takes good care of you at home, doesn't she?"
    4. "Are you feeling guilty because your parent has pneumonia?"

31. A client has pregnancy-induced hypertension (PIH). In planning care for this client prior to delivery, the most essential nursing order is to:

    1. Assess fluid balance hourly and maintain optimum placental perfusion.
    2. Monitor urine output and assure a brief rest period every shift.
    3. Check the blood pressure before and after each time the client is out of bed.
    4. Observe for amount of edema and provide for diversionary activities.

32. A client sustained a T-4 spinal cord injury. While doing morning assessments four weeks post-injury, the nurse discovers the client's BP is 280/140 and the client is complaining of nasal stuffiness and a severe, pounding headache. The first nursing action is to:

    1. Sit the client upright.
    2. Call the physician.
    3. Check the client's bladder for distension.
    4. Administer the prescribed antihypertensive.

33. A client is in the hospital with renal failure and is on fluid restriction. The nurse knows it would be inappropriate to:

    1. Furnish a variety of fluids in small containers.
    2. Inform the client and family about the restriction.
    3. Allow the client to help keep a record of oral intake.
    4. Provide fluids only during meal times.

34. The physician has ordered a client to be discharged on a 2,000 calorie-per-day diet. What is the most important nursing action in developing a teaching plan for this client's diet?

    1. Obtain sample menus from the dietitian to give to the client.
    2. Ask the client to identify the types of foods usually eaten and preferred.
    3. Tell the client that all of the client's previous eating habits will have to be changed.
    4. Advise the client to buy only dietetic foods.

35. An eight-year-old client is admitted to the hospital with a diagnosis of acute rheumatic fever. Immediately after admission, which nursing assessment is most important?

    1. Auscultation of the rate and characteristics of heart sounds.
    2. Determining the location and severity of joint pain.
    3. Identifying the degree of anxiety related to the diagnosis.
    4. Determining the family's emotional and financial needs.

36. A client recently diagnosed with multiple sclerosis questions the nurse concerning the usual course of the disease. What would be the most appropriate response by the nurse?

    1. "Each client is different. We cannot tell what will happen."
    2. "I can see that you are worried, but it's too soon to predict what will happen."
    3. "Usually, acute episodes are followed by remissions, which may last a long time."
    4. "It's too early to think about the future; let's focus on the present and go day-by-day."

37. While transferring a client with left-leg weakness from the bed to a wheelchair, the priority nursing action is to:

    1. Have the seat of the wheelchair at a right angle to the bed.
    2. Lock the wheels on the bed and the wheelchair.
    3. Allow the client to do as much as possible to increase sense of independence.
    4. Tell the client to lock the hands around the nurse's neck to provide a sense of security.

38. A nurse enters the room and finds the parent of a child diagnosed with leukemia crying. The child is currently receiving chemotherapy. The parent says, "I just can't believe my child is going to lose all that beautiful blonde hair!" Which response by the nurse is most therapeutic?

    1. "Sometimes the hair only thins."
    2. "You're feeling a lot of loss right now."
    3. "Remember, hair loss means the chemotherapy is working!"
    4. "Kids love to wear the special baseball caps we have."

39. A client says to the nurse, "I am so frustrated with having five kids. My husband won't do anything to help keep me from getting pregnant." The initial nursing action is to:

    1. Refer the client and spouse to family planning services.
    2. Find out if the client could use a contraceptive that would not involve her husband.
    3. Inquire what the client means by "being frustrated."
    4. Ask the client if her husband is interested in birth control.

40. **An adult client is diagnosed with pneumonia and is being treated with penicillin G sodium 3 million units IV every four hours. When completing the drug history, it is especially important for the nurse to assess the client for allergies to:**

    1. Antituberculars.
    2. Calcium channel blockers.
    3. Aminoglycosides.
    4. Cephalosporins.

41. **A client is gravida 5 para 4. During admission, the nurse assesses that contractions are occurring every two minutes and are lasting approximately 45 seconds. The client sayshas been in labor for approximately 10 hours. The priority assessment the nurse needs to make at this time is:**

    1. Time the client last ate.
    2. Cervical dilatation.
    3. Allergies to medications.
    4. Vital signs.

42. **A client is admitted to the hospital at 38 weeks gestation with a large amount of bright red vaginal bleeding. A diagnosis of partial abruptio placenta is made on the fetal monitor, and her vital signs are: FH 138 regular, BP 98/52, pulse 118, respirations 24, temperature 97.6 degrees F. Assuming all of the following are ordered by the physician, the nurse should give first priority to which nursing action?**

    1. Abdominal-perineal prep.
    2. Insert Foley catheter.
    3. Sign informed consent for surgery.
    4. Start an IV.

43. **A 15-year-old female client is being seen in the family planning clinic. She says to the nurse that she is nervous and has never had a pelvic examination before. The appropriate response by the nurse is:**

    1. "All you have to do is relax."
    2. "It is only slightly uncomfortable."
    3. "What part of the exam makes you nervous?"
    4. "If you want birth control pills, then a pelvic exam is required."

44. **If a nurse discovered a fire in a client's room, the first nursing action would be to:**

    1. Pull the fire alarm and notify the hospital operator.
    2. Close fire doors and client room doors.
    3. Remove the client from the room.
    4. Place moist towels or blankets at the threshold of the door of the room with the fire.

45. **In assessing an adult client with diabetes mellitus, the nurse identifies an unexpected finding as:**

    1. Possible increased body weight.
    2. Increased urinary output.
    3. Periods of polydypsia.
    4. Altered heart rate and rhythm.

46. **A client, who is paralyzed from the waist down, is to be up in a chair three times a day. What is the best nursing approach when transferring the client from a bed into a wheelchair?**

    1. Place the wheelchair close to the foot of the bed.
    2. Utilize the principles of body mechanics while providing a safe transfer for the client.
    3. Slide the client to the edge of the bed, keeping the nurse's back straight, and use a rocking motion to pull the client.
    4. Place the nurse's arms under the client's axillae from the back of the client.

47. **A client puts the call light on and indicates a need to urinate. The client has had a Foley catheter in place since surgery two days ago. The nurse's initial action is to:**

    1. Remind the client that because a Foley catheter is in place, the client does not need to go to the bathroom.
    2. Replace the Foley catheter with a new catheter.
    3. Explain to the client that the urge to void is a common occurrence for clients who have urinary catheters.
    4. Check the catheter and tubing for kinks and note the urine output in the drainage bag.

48. **A 49-year-old client has been diagnosed with iron deficiency anemia. When teaching the client about diet, the nurse should recommend an increased intake of:**

    1. Fresh fruits.
    2. Milk and cheese.
    3. Organ meats.
    4. Whole grain breads.

49. **A client is to have a nasogastric tube inserted because of a bowel obstruction. The nurse explains the procedure and is about to begin the insertion when the client says, "No way! You are not putting that hose down my throat. Get away from me." The best nursing response is:**

    1. "You have the right to refuse treatment. Why don't you talk to your doctor about it?"
    2. "Something is upsetting you. Can you tell me what it is?"
    3. "What exactly do you feel about this 'hose'?"
    4. "It'll be easier for you to just get it over with. It only gets harder if you get worked up over it and you won't get better without this tube."

50. The nurse tells a client that the doctor has ordered an intravenous line to be started. The client appears to be upset, but says nothing to the nurse. Which is the best nursing response to this situation?

    1. "Do you have any questions about the procedure?"
    2. "The doctor wants you to have antibiotics, and this method eliminates getting frequent injections."
    3. "What is there about this procedure that concerns you?"
    4. "It only hurts a little bit. It'll be over before you know it."

51. A client shows the nurse the result of a recent tuberculin skin test. The site is red and swollen. The nurse interprets this as the:

    1. Client has active tuberculosis.
    2. Client has a history of tuberculosis.
    3. Tubercle bacillus is in the active pulmonary stage of tuberculosis.
    4. Client has had contact with the tubercle bacillus.

52. A client is in the hospital and has weakness on the left side because of a stroke. The client becomes upset when eating because liquids drool out of the weak side of the mouth. What nursing intervention would be most appropriate?

    1. Providing only pureed and solid foods to prevent drooling.
    2. Letting a member of the family assist with the client's feedings.
    3. Teaching the client how to drink fluids on the unaffected side to prevent drooling.
    4. Having the client use a syringe to squirt liquids into the back of the mouth.

53. A 10-year-old client is in sickle cell crisis. Which nursing action is contraindicated?

    1. Administer oxygen via nasal cannula as prescribed.
    2. Encourage the client to increase oral fluid intake.
    3. Administer narcotics only for very severe pain.
    4. Encourage as much exercise as possible during the crisis.

54. A client has sustained a basal skull fracture and the nurse notices drainage from the client's right nostril. The priority nursing action is to:

    l. Notify the physician.
    2. Suction the nostril.
    3. Test the drainage for glucose.
    4. Ask the client to blow the nose.

55. If verapamil hydrochloride (Calan) is administered with propranolol (Inderal), the nurse should monitor the client closely for signs of:

    1. Hypertension.
    2. Increased peripheral resistance.
    3. Bradycardia and heart failure.
    4. Diarrhea.

56. In assessing a client after a bronchoscopy, the nurse would give immediate attention to:

    1. Blood-tinged mucous.
    2. Complaints of hoarseness when speaking.
    3. Irritation and discomfort when swallowing.
    4. Difficulty breathing.

57. The nurse is caring for a client who had abdominal surgery two days ago. Which assessment data requires immediate action by the nurse?

    1. A urinary drainage bag with 100 mL in a two-hour period.
    2. A wound dressing with thick, light green drainage.
    3. A blood pressure reading of 98/66.
    4. Shallow respirations, with a rate of 26.

58. A depressed client attends a client education class on the topic of depression and learn about the behaviors that could indicate a recurrence of depression. To evaluate the effectiveness of the teaching, the nurse asks the client to identify the indications of recurrence of depression. Which behavior or manifestation, if named by the client, would indicate to the nurse the need for further instruction?

    1. Psychomotor retardation.
    2. Grandiosity.
    3. Self-devaluation.
    4. Insomnia.

59. An 18-month-old child is admitted for a surgical repair of the cleft palate. The child returns from the operating room supine, with an IV and a mist tent on room air. Which is the priority nursing action?

    1. Medicate for pain.
    2. Check the IV for signs of infiltration.
    3. Turn the child on the side.
    4. Review the postoperative orders.

60. A male nurse receives a doctor's order to catheterize one of his female clients. The client says, "I'm not going to allow a male nurse to catheterize me." The appropriate response by the nurse is:

    1. "Your doctor is a male. Would you let him catheterize you?"
    2. "I've done this many times with no problems."
    3. "You can explain to your doctor why the catheter wasn't inserted."
    4. "You appear to be upset. Let me find a female nurse to help with the procedure."

61. A confused elderly client is found wandering around the ward wearing a bathrobe and cotton socks. The client is bumping into walls while walking. At this time, the nurse should:

1. Bring the client's shoes and help the client put them on.
2. Accompany the client back to the room and obtain a baseline assessment.
3. Ask the client to return to the room and rest until feeling better.
4. Tell the client to be careful of any wet spots on the floor.

62. **A conscious client is brought to the emergency room after an automobile accident. A physical examination and x-rays reveal a transection of the spinal cord at T-4. The nurse should give the highest priority to which information? The client:**

1. Has an allergy to iodine.
2. Last voided seven hours ago.
3. Smokes two packs of cigarettes a day.
4. Is menstruating.

63. **A female client is taking ampicillin (Amcill) and birth control pills containing estrogen. What information should the nurse provide?**

1. Take both medications with breakfast to avoid gastric upset.
2. When used together, serum potassium levels may rise.
3. The effectiveness of the birth control pills may be reduced while the client is taking ampicillin.
4. Urticaria is much more common when antibiotics are given with other drugs.

64. **A client is admitted to the hospital for surgery after finding a lump in his right testicle. He asks the nurse, "Do you think the doctor will find cancer?" What is the best nursing response?**

1. "Most lumps found in the testicles are benign."
2. "It must be difficult for you not to know what the doctor will find."
3. "I think that you should discuss this with your doctor."
4. "It might be, but the doctor won't know until the surgery is performed."

65. **A client's psychiatrist orders lithium (Lithane) four times daily. When administering medications on the sixth day, the nurse notes that the client's laboratory report indicates a serum lithium level of 1.0 mEq/liter. Based on this lab report, the most appropriate nursing action at this time is to:**

1. Withhold the next dose of lithium and notify the psychiatrist.
2. Ask that the laboratory test be repeated.
3. Assess the client for possible toxic effects.
4. Administer the next dose of lithium as ordered.

66. **A client is seen in the clinic in the 28th week of gestation. Her blood pressure is 160/100 and she has 2+ protein in her urine. Her doctor recommends hospitalization. Because each available room on the unit is a semiprivate room, the client must share a room. The nurse knows the appropriate roommate for this client is a:**

1. 20-year-old primigravida who enjoys loud rock-and-roll music.
2. 32-year-old multigravida who enjoys reading romance novels.
3. 24-year-old C-section who watches soap operas and game shows on TV.
4. 22-year-old primigravida who has many visitors during the afternoon and evening.

67. **A client asks the nurse how relaxation techniques will help reduce gastric pain. The client asks, "Can't I just take the cimetidine (Tagamet) that my physician has prescribed?" In responding to this question, the nurse is guided by the knowledge that:**

1. Gastric ulcer is a stress-related illness, and the client's stress levels and emotional issues are contributing to the exacerbation of the manifestations.
2. The client is in denial, because the client is refusing to acknowledge the role stress plays in the progress of this illness.
3. Gastric ulcer and other psychosomatic illnesses are caused by stress and cannot be cured with only medical or surgical treatments.
4. The client is displaying the "typical ulcer personality" of a competitive, aggressive person who is defending against unresolved dependency needs.

68. **A six-week-old infant with AIDS is being prepared for discharge. The infant's primary caregiver is the grandmother. Which statement by the grandmother would alert the nurse to a need for further instruction?**

1. "I know that handwashing is an important preventative measure."
2. "I'll use disposable diapers, discarding them in separate plastic bags."
3. "Blood spills should be washed up immediately with hot soapy water."
4. "Gloves should be worn by all persons changing the baby's diapers."

69. **The most important nursing goal for a client who is admitted with an acute exacerbation of ulcerative colitis is to:**

1. Provide emotional support.
2. Prevent skin breakdown.
3. Maintain fluid and electrolyte balance.
4. Promote physical rest.

70. The nurse observes an elderly client trying to climb over the side rails of the bed. The nurse is placing a vest restraint on the client when the daughter arrives and says to the nurse, "My parent does not need to be tied down in bed. I've been taking care of my parent for years, and my parent hasn't fallen out of bed yet." The initial response by the nurse is:

1. "I just saw your parent trying to climb over the side rails. Since I am concerned about your parent falling and getting hurt, I think this is best for safety."
2. "Tell me how you managed to care for your parent at home."
3. "Hospital policy requires restraint vests on clients who are at risk for falling. I just saw your parent trying to climb over the rails. You don't want your parent to get hurt, do you?"
4. "The elderly may become confused in an unfamiliar place and do things they wouldn't do at home. It is difficult to see your parent restrained. While you are with your parent, the restraints can be off. Let me know when you are ready to leave."

71. The nurse is caring for a client who is recovering from surgery. The client has a urinary catheter in place that needs to be irrigated. The nurse knows the correct approach to prevent injury to the mucosa of the bladder is:

1. Gently compress the ball of the syringe to instill the irrigating solution.
2. Quickly instill the irrigating solution, using some pressure to loosen any clots or mucous.
3. After instilling the solution, apply gentle pressure to remove the irrigating solution from the bladder.
4. Place a sterile cap on the end of the drainage tubing to protect it from contamination.

72. A client is admitted to the hospital because of extreme weight loss. It is noted on the admission assessment that the client feels overweight at 88 pounds. What aspect of care should the nurse consider the first priority for this client's care?

1. Assessing the client's nutritional status.
2. Obtaining a psychiatric consult.
3. Planning a therapeutic diet for the client.
4. Talking to family members to find out more about the client's self-concept.

73. A client is hospitalized for a closed reduction of a fractured femur and application of a cast. A vital nursing action in the care of this client is to:

1. Perform neurovascular checks of the extremities.
2. Use the palms of the hands when moving an extremity with a wet cast.
3. Provide an instrument for the client to scratch the itching areas of skin under the cast.
4. Petal the edges of the cast to provide smooth edges.

74. After detoxification, a client begins the rehabilitation phase of treatment. The client tells the nurse, "I cannot imagine living my life without alcohol." The nurse's best response is based on the knowledge that the client:

1. Will be more successful if the client focuses on goals for short periods of time.
2. Is likely to drink again when under stress.
3. Will not be successful if the client is not strongly motivated.
4. May require treatment with Antabuse to maintain sobriety.

75. While performing a vaginal exam on an obstetrical client, the nurse notes a glistening white cord in the vagina. The first nursing action is to:

1. Return to the nurses' station to place an emergency call to the physician.
2. Start oxygen at six to 10 liters, and assess the client's vital signs.
3. Cover the cord with a sterile, moist saline dressing.
4. Apply manual pressure on the presenting part and have the mother get into a knee-chest position.

76. A client is in the hospital and has just found out that the parent died of a heart attack. The client is crying and has the face buried in a pillow. The most therapeutic nursing response at this time is to:

1. Return in fifteen minutes to see how the client is doing.
2. Sit with the client for a little while.
3. Tell the client that things will feel better in the morning.
4. Share with the client that the nurse knows just how the client feels because the nurse's parent recently died.

77. A client with asthma is receiving an oxygen concentration of 35%. The nurse knows that achievement of the therapeutic goal of this treatment is best demonstrated by:

1. Absence of adventitious breath sounds.
2. PaO_2 92.
3. Heart rate increase of 25 beats/min.
4. Bicarbonate level of 25 mEq/liter.

78. The primary nurse learns that an obsessive-compulsive client has a full set of dentures because the client's brushing rituals eroded all of the tooth enamel. The client also brushes the tongue several times a day, and has developed several ulcerations on it. The initial priority in the nursing care plan for this client is for the client to:

1. Eliminate the brushing and mouth care rituals.
2. Verbalize the underlying cause of this behavior.
3. Seek out the nurse when feeling anxious.
4. Reestablish healthy tissue in the mouth and tongue.

79. **The nurse is informed during report that a postoperative client has not voided for eight hours. The initial nursing action is to:**

   1. Assist the client to the bathroom.
   2. Place the client on a bed pan and pour warm water over the perineum.
   3. Palpate and percuss the client's bladder.
   4. Catheterize the client.

80. **A three-year-old is being admitted with nephrotic syndrome. The best roommate the nurse can select for this client is:**

   1. A 16-year-old recovering post-operatively from a ruptured appendix.
   2. An eight-year-old with leukemia.
   3. Another toddler with rheumatic fever.
   4. No roommate because isolation is required.

81. **A client is to receive antibiotics. The priority nursing action when preparing to administer this medication is to:**

   1. Determine if the client has any allergies.
   2. Determine the route of administration.
   3. Check the client's name band.
   4. Check the dosage against the physician's order.

82. **Before administering lithium, the nurse checks the client's latest lab report for the serum lithium level and notes a level of 1.2 mEq/L. What is the best action for the nurse to take next?**

   1. Administer the next prescribed dose of lithium.
   2. Suggest the blood test be repeated.
   3. Withhold the next dose of lithium and notify the psychiatrist of the lab results.
   4. Ask the client how he is feeling, to identify any untoward effects.

83. **A client is admitted to the psychiatric unit with a diagnosis of acute depression. After being hospitalized for a few weeks, the client says to the nurse, "I'm a terrible person, and I should be dead." The nurse understands that the initial response would be:**

   1. "That is why you are here. We are trying to help you with your bad feelings."
   2. "Feeling that way must be awful. What makes you feel so terrible?"
   3. "Feeling like a terrible person is part of your illness. As you get better, those feelings will lessen."
   4. "You are not terrible. You are not a bad person."

84. **The nurse in a long-term care facility finds an elderly client on the floor. After having the client examined by the physician, the most important nursing action is to:**

   1. Call the family to stay with the client.
   2. Provide for the safety and protection of the client.
   3. Apply wrist and leg restraints to prevent the client from falling out of bed.
   4. Obtain an order for medication to sedate the client.

85. **A client was admitted one week ago with a diagnosis of schizophrenia, paranoid type. Since admission, the client has had several verbal outbursts of anger but has not been violent. A staff member tells the nurse that the client is pacing up and down the hall very rapidly and muttering in an angry manner. The initial nursing action is to:**

   1. Prepare an intramuscular injection of haloperidol (Haldol) to give the client p.r.n.
   2. Observe the behavior and approach the client in a non-threatening manner.
   3. Gather several staff members and approach the client together.
   4. Contact the client's psychiatrist and request an order to place the client in seclusion.

86. **Betamethasone (Celestone) is administered to a client at 30 weeks gestation to reduce the risk of respiratory distress syndrome (RDS) in the neonate. The infant is born after two injections are given. In planning nursing care for the infant, which finding should be anticipated as a result of the administration of betamethasone to the mother?**

   1. Rapid pulse rate.
   2. Sternal retractions.
   3. Hypoglycemia.
   4. Hypothermia.

87. **In preparing to begin an aminophylline (Phyllocontin) infusion, the best nursing approach would be:**

   1. Preparing a solution containing enough drug to last 24 hours.
   2. Obtaining an infusion pump to regulate the flow of the drug.
   3. Inserting a large IV catheter to assure adequate dilution.
   4. Initiating measurement of intake and output to detect fluid retention.

88. **A client is being given an aminoglycoside for a bacterial infection. The nurse can aid in minimizing the risk of aminoglycoside toxicity by:**

   1. Weighing the client daily.
   2. Encouraging the client to drink at least 2,000 mL of fluids daily.
   3. Monitoring blood pressure prior to drug administration.
   4. Instructing the client to take the medicine with food.

89. A client is hospitalized for gastrointestinal bleeding and is being treated with temazepam (Restoril). After the physician examined the client, the nurse noted the physician wrote an order for the client to begin taking amitriptyline (Elavil). The initial action by the nurse is to:

    1. Revise the client's medication schedule so that the Elavil is administered during the day and the Restoril at bedtime.
    2. Monitor the client's vital signs closely.
    3. Question the physician about administering both Elavil and Restoril to the client.
    4. Assess the client for manifestations of depression.

90. The nurse is caring for a client with a myocardial infarction who is taking chlorothiazide (Diuril) and digoxin (Lanoxin). The most appropriate diet for the nurse to include in this client's nursing care is a diet:

    1. Low in sodium and saturated fats, high in potassium.
    2. Low in unsaturated fats, sodium, and potassium.
    3. High in potassium, Vitamin C, and protein.
    4. Low in sodium and saturated and unsaturated fats.

91. The nurse is caring for a client with diabetes who is currently taking cephalexin (Keflex). The nurse should advise the client that:

    1. Clinitest or copper sulfate urine glucose tests give false positive results.
    2. Blood sugar may drop without warning.
    3. A source of sugar should always be carried with the client.
    4. A MedicAlert bracelet should always be worn.

92. An elderly client is admitted to the psychiatric unit for a diagnostic work-up because of increased forgetfulness and disorientation at home. The client has been taking lorazepam (Ativan) 0.5 mg p.r.n. to control restlessness. In planning nursing care for this client, it would be unnecessary to include close observation for:

    1. Orthostatic hypotension.
    2. Increased anxiety.
    3. Hyperexcitation.
    4. Hallucinations.

93. A client with chronic emphysema is taking theophylline (Theo-Dur) at home. During the home care nurse's visit, which statement by the client would warrant immediate action?

    1. "I just lie awake at night, worrying about the medical bills."
    2. "I must have the flu. I was vomiting all night."
    3. "I don't have my usual appetite. Nothing tastes good to me."
    4. "I feel better if I have a big glass of milk with my pill."

94. A client is admitted to the psychiatric unit with a diagnosis of acute psychotic reaction. Because of extreme agitation, the client is started on chlorpromazine (Thorazine) 100 mg t.i.d. After three days, the client is much calmer and the nurse begins to teach the client about this medication. Which statement by the nurse is most appropriate?

    1. "This medication is a sedative to calm you down."
    2. "This medication acts on the chemical regulators in your brain to help control your manifestations."
    3. "This medication will cure your disorder."
    4. "We do not know how this medication works, but we do know it will help you control your behavior."

95. A client is to have surgery the next day to create an ileal conduit and is receiving neomycin sulfate (Mycifradin Sulfate). The nurse's best explanation to the client for receiving neomycin preoperatively is that it:

    1. Suppresses intestinal bacteria preoperatively, to decrease the risk of postoperative infection.
    2. Decreases the number of pathogenic bacteria and decreases the number of loose stools.
    3. Sterilizes the bowel and prevents the risk of serious postoperative complications.
    4. Prevents auditory impairment and nephrotoxicity during the postoperative period.

96. A client is admitted with pneumocystis carinii pneumonitis. The physician prescribes sulfamethoxazole trimethoprim (Bactrim), and a Foley catheter is inserted to monitor urinary output. Which nursing intervention would be most effective in reducing the risk of crystalluria secondary to sulfonamide therapy?

    1. Encouraging fluid intake to 3,000 mL/24 hours.
    2. Irrigating the Foley catheter with normal saline every eight hours.
    3. Monitoring specific gravity of urine every eight hours.
    4. Providing foods and fluids likely to maintain an acidic pH of the urine.

97. A client is to receive IM methylergonovine (Methergine). In caring for the client, the nurse knows the administration of IM Methergine is contraindicated in a client:

    1. Who is experiencing boggy fundus one hour after a vaginal delivery.
    2. With a large amount of vaginal bleeding following an abortion at 16 weeks.
    3. With a history of previous postpartum hemorrhage in the recovery room.
    4. Who has not delivered the placenta 20 minutes following the birth of the baby.

98. A client is receiving propranolol (Inderal) for anxiety. In reviewing the client's discharge plans, the nurse needs to emphasize that Inderal:

   1. Should be discontinued by gradually tapering it off over time.
   2. Should not be taken during pregnancy.
   3. Is contraindicated for clients with asthma.
   4. Is a safe medication with no known adverse effects.

99. A client has been taking trifluoperazine (Stelazine) for five years to control paranoid thoughts. When the client's sibling comes to visit, the sibling tells the nurse, "I believe that all psychiatric medications are a form of 'chemical mind control'." The nurse's best response to the sibling will incorporate the information that antipsychotic medications:

   1. Act directly on specific neurotransmitters in the brain to control the client's psychotic manifestations.
   2. Act to sedate the client, therefore preventing the client from engaging in behavior that may cause difficulty.
   3. Are a cure for psychotic disorders, like schizophrenic reactions, and are therefore an important part of the client's treatment plan.
   4. Have been in use for close to 30 years and are safe and effective drugs for clients who have problems like this client's.

100. Which measure would the nurse select as providing the most accurate determination of renal impairment secondary to administration of amphotericin B (Fungizone)?

   1. Intake and output.
   2. Daily weights.
   3. Serum creatinine levels.
   4. Serial potassium levels.

CONGRATULATIONS!
You have reached the end of the Final Exam. Now, turn to Chapter Eleven to score your exam, assess your progress, and read rationales.

NOTES

Chapter 11

ANSWERS AND ANALYSES

Before you turn the page and look for the answers to the Final Exam, read the following reminders. And remember, the more test questions you answer during your review practice sessions, the better you will become at taking this kind of exam. Practice makes perfect!

Making the Most of Your Final Exam Results

- If you answered a question incorrectly, **determine whether you did not know the material or just misread the question.** If you misread a question, identify the **critical element** that was overlooked. You need to minimize the questions you are answering incorrectly because of misreading!

- When you review the answers to the questions—using either this chapter or the Answers and Analyses post-test section on the disk—be sure to read the rationales: You might have answered a question correctly using an incorrect rationale! (In your practice sessions, always review the rationales.)

- Try to determine how many questions you answered correctly **by using one of the three test-taking strategies.** When you are unsure of an answer, eliminating incorrect options and using test-taking strategies can increase your score dramatically!

- Use the Assessment Scale on the following page to assess your progress.

Assessment Scale

Score	Recommendation
Less than 65%	OOPS! Don't get discouraged! Spend some time reviewing the basic concepts and strategies in Chapters Three and Four, and try again.
65-75%	Good work. Try reviewing the "Test-Taking Tips" and "Points to Remember," and keep practicing.
75-85%	Very good. You are becoming a good strategist! Keep answering practice questions until the exam.
85%+	Superior work! Continue to apply these principles and try to ace the exam!

- After calculating your score and analyzing your answers, you should **continue to practice answering questions and assessing your progress on a daily basis.** This is especially important for NCLEX-RN candidates! But nursing students should continue to practice these new test-taking skills, too.

- If you are an NCLEX-RN candidate and were not able to use the computer disk enclosed with this book, be sure to plan some time on a computer in your learning lab to practice taking a computerized exam. You might also wish to use some of the other NCLEX-RN review materials, including comprehensive review manuals, audio or video tapes, and especially Q&A books and software. MEDS, Inc. offers a comprehensive Q&A review, which uses the same Personal Performance Analysis as the disk accompanying this book. The more test questions you answer, the better!

We hope *Test Question Logic (TQLogic™) for the NCLEX-RN Exam* has revolutionized your approach to taking an exam, and to studying and reviewing material. You have acquired an important new professional skill.

GOOD LUCK IN YOUR COURSES AND ON THE NCLEX-RN!

1. **A nurse visits a client at home one week following discharge after a myocardial infarction. The client is taking chlorothiazide (Diuril) 500 mg daily and digoxin (Lanoxin) 0.25 mg daily. The nurse should give top priority to assessing the client's knowledge of:**

   1. Sources of potassium.
   2. Sources of sodium.
   3. Activity restrictions.
   4. Signs of a heart attack.

   1. ***CORRECT. Because the client is taking both Diuril and Lanoxin, the nurse should focus on the client's knowledge of sources of potassium. Diuril depletes potassium. If the potassium level is too low, digoxin toxicity may lead to serious cardiac arrhythmias. This is the top priority because lack of understanding may cause a life-threatening situation.***
   2. *INCORRECT. The client is probably on a sodium restricted diet. Too much sodium will increase the cardiac workload. The nurse should assess the client's knowledge of sources of sodium but based on the information provided in the case scenario, this is not the top priority.*
   3. *INCORRECT. The client will increase activity gradually while recuperating from the myocardial infarction. The nurse should assess the client's knowledge of activity restrictions but based on the information provided in the case scenario, this is not the top priority.*
   4. *INCORRECT. The nurse should assess the client's knowledge of the signs of another heart attack but based on the information provided in the case scenario, this is not the top priority.*

2. **An adolescent client is to have a water system heating device (K-Pad) applied to a pulled muscle. The client tells the nurse that the device does not feel very warm. The most appropriate nursing action is to:**

   1. Explain to the client that these heating devices never feel hot.
   2. Check the temperature setting on the heating unit and feel the pad for warmth.
   3. Call the appropriate repair department and have them fix the unit.
   4. Turn the temperature up on the unit if it doesn't feel warm enough to the client.

   1. *INCORRECT. Although these heating units do feel warm and not hot, the unit may not be at a therapeutic temperature, and should be assessed to see if it is working properly. You are looking for the most appropriate nursing action. TEST-TAKING TIP: Remember the nursing process—assess first.*
   2. ***CORRECT. The nurse should check that the device is set to the temperature recommended by the manufacturer. The nurse should also assess whether the pad feels warm. TEST-TAKING TIP: Remember the nursing process—assess first.***

3. *INCORRECT. The unit may not be malfunctioning. It should be assessed by the nurse before any other action is taken. If the unit is malfunctioning, it should be replaced with another unit, and the malfunctioning unit should be sent to the repair department. TEST-TAKING TIP: Remember the nursing process—assess first.*
4. *INCORRECT. The temperature should not be set above the recommended setting, to avoid causing a burn to the client. TEST-TAKING TIP: Remember the nursing process—assess first.*

3. **A client who weighs 288 pounds says to the nurse, "I'm going to have surgery to have my stomach stapled so I can lose weight. I've tried everything else, and nothing seems to work." Which response by the nurse would be therapeutic?**

   1. "That's a pretty drastic measure. Are you sure that is what you want to do?"
   2. "I hear that the surgery is only a temporary measure, and if you have the staples removed, you will only gain the weight back again."
   3. "It must be difficult to be overweight and not able to lose weight. What does your spouse think about the surgery?"
   4. "Can you tell me about the possible consequences and side effects of this type of surgery?"

   1. *INCORRECT. This response by the nurse is judgmental and questions the decision made by the client. There is no encouragement from the nurse that promotes further communication from the client. This is not a therapeutic nursing response.*

   > **TEST-TAKING TIP:** This is an implementation question that asks for an appropriate response by the nurse. In communication questions, look for an option that uses a therapeutic communication tool and addresses the client's feelings and concerns.

   2. *INCORRECT. This may or may not be an accurate statement, but it does not promote therapeutic communication. The client is frustrated about the weight and needs to express these feelings. This response indicates to the client that the situation is hopeless. TEST-TAKING TIP: This is an implementation question that asks for an appropriate response by the nurse. In communication questions, look for an option that uses a therapeutic communication tool and addresses the client's feelings and concerns.*
   3. *INCORRECT. This response is only half correct. The first part uses the therapeutic communication tool of empathy, but the second part (asking about the spouse's feelings) blocks communication by focusing on an inappropriate person. TEST-TAKING TIP: Starting an incorrect answer off with correct buzzwords is a common ploy in distracters, which is why memorization alone is worthless for the NCLEX-RN. Recognizing buzzwords without understanding the theory behind them and its proper application can lead the nurse candidate to choose distracters like this one.*

4. CORRECT. This response is therapeutic because it asks for clarification of the client's understanding of the surgery and promotes further communication.

4. The nurse finds an elderly client standing in a puddle of water in the unit's hallway. The nurse does not know this client. What should the nurse do first?

1. Ask the client's name and room number.
2. Wipe up the water until the floor is completely dry.
3. Call the supervisor for assistance in identifying the client.
4. Have the client wait in the lounge until security arrives.

1. *INCORRECT. The issue in this question is the puddle of water on the floor. The water on the floor threatens the safety of the client and others on the unit. After eliminating the safety hazard, the nurse can identify the client and assist the client back to the proper room.*

2. CORRECT. The issue in this question is the puddle of water on the floor. The water on the floor threatens the safety of the client and others on the unit. The nurse's first action should be to alleviate the safety hazard by wiping up the water. Maslow's hierarchy of needs indicates that, when no physiological need exists, safety needs should receive priority.

> **TEST-TAKING TIP:** The idea of water on the floor is repeated in this option. The test-taking strategy of looking for similar words or phrases in the question would identify this option as a possible answer if you were unsure of the best response.

3. *INCORRECT. The issue in this question is the puddle of water on the floor. The water on the floor threatens the safety of the client and others on the unit. After eliminating the safety hazard, the nurse can identify the client and assist the client back to the proper room.*

4. *INCORRECT. The issue in this question is the puddle of water on the floor. The water on the floor threatens the safety of the client and others on the unit. Asking the client to wait in the lounge until security arrives does not ensure safety. Someone may still slip on the puddle of water and injure themselves.*

5. The nurse caring for a client on the evening before a scheduled left below-the-knee amputation provides preoperative teaching, including deep breathing and coughing. Which question would be most helpful for the nurse to ask the client to evaluate the effectiveness of the preoperative teaching?

1. "Do you understand what we have just discussed about deep breathing and coughing?"
2. "Do you think that you will need to have a sedative to help you sleep tonight?"
3. "Will you demonstrate for me the correct method of deep breathing and coughing?"
4. "Do you have any questions concerning your scheduled surgical procedure?"

1. *INCORRECT. This is not the best option. This question asks the client about the content of the preoperative teaching in the form of a closed question, which requires only a "yes" or "no" answer. The client could answer "yes" regardless of the true state of understanding. This is not the best question to ask.*

2. *INCORRECT. The test question asked you to select a question that the nurse should ask to evaluate preoperative teaching. In this option, the nurse is asking about the need for a sedative, not about the client's understanding of preoperative teaching. Although the question is an appropriate question for the nurse to ask at this time, it is not the correct answer because it does not relate to the issue in the question.*

3. CORRECT. This question asks the client about the content of the preoperative teaching. In addition, the question requests a return demonstration of deep breathing and coughing. If the preoperative teaching has been effective, the client will be able to do the return demonstration. If additional teaching is required, the client will be unable to do the return demonstration properly. This is the best question for evaluating the effectiveness of preoperative teaching.

4. *INCORRECT. This question is an appropriate question for the nurse to ask at this time. It is not the correct answer, however, because the stem of this test question asks you to select a question that the nurse should ask to evaluate preoperative teaching. Here, the nurse is asking about the client's understanding of the surgical procedure. The client's questions concerning the surgical procedure should be referred to the doctor.*

6. The nurse is conducting a preoperative interview three days prior to admitting a seven-year-old client for a tonsillectomy. The client's parent requests information to prepare the child for hospitalization. The nurse knows that the child was hospitalized last year for a fractured femur. Which nursing actions would best meet this child's needs for preparation?

1. Suggest a role play and provide materials.
2. Remind the child of the experience of the past hospitalization.
3. Read the child a story about another child having a similar operation.
4. Tell the child the appointment is only to have the throat checked.

1. CORRECT. This best meets the child's needs because concrete experiences are the most meaningful learning for the school age child. This is the rationale for pediatric orientation programs. Even if there is inadequate time for the client to participate in such a program, a shortened version with practice with a mask and other equipment in a non-threatening environment would be helpful.

2. *INCORRECT. This is not the best action because past experiences, especially traumatic ones, may not have been positive.*

3. INCORRECT. This isn't the best response. This is somewhat abstract, and abstract thinking is not highly developed in the seven-year-old child.

4. INCORRECT. This is an inappropriate action. The nurse should never lie to a child. This is inappropriate under any circumstances.

7. A client is admitted to the hospital in respiratory distress. The doctor orders oxygen via mask and the client to be placed in Fowler's position. Which nursing action is most important for this client at this time?

1. Support and align the hands with the forearms.
2. Use handrolls.
3. Raise the head of the bed to allow for greater lung expansion.
4. Support the feet at right angles to the lower legs.

1. INCORRECT. This option does not address the issue of the question, which is a nursing action to counter respiratory distress. Supporting and aligning the hands prevents potential contractures of the wrist; however, it is not the most important action at this time.

2. INCORRECT. This option does not address the issue of the question, which is a nursing action to counter respiratory distress. Handrolls aid in preventing contractures by maintaining the fingers and thumbs in a functional position; however, it is not the most important nursing action at this time.

3. CORRECT. The elevation of the head of the bed allows for greater lung expansion and decreased respiratory effort. This option correctly addresses the issue of the question, which is a nursing action to counter respiratory distress.

> **TEST-TAKING TIP:** The similar words "respiratory" and "lung expansion" are found in the question and this option, respectively. The test-taking strategy of looking for similar words or phrases in the question would identify this option as a possible answer if you were unsure of the best response.

4. INCORRECT. This option does not address the issue of the question, which is a nursing action to counter respiratory distress. Supporting the feet prevents foot drop and contractures at the ankle; however, this is not the most important action at this time.

8. A 23-year-old gravida 1, para 0 is admitted to the hospital at 38 weeks gestation with pregnancy induced hypertension (PIH). Which finding would the nurse identify as inconsistent with the admitting diagnosis?

1. 3+ protein in the urine.
2. Deep tendon reflexes of +1.
3. Blood pressure of 148/98.
4. 1+ pitting sacral edema.

1. INCORRECT. Manifestations of PIH include proteinuria, edema, and elevated blood pressure. A finding of 3+ protein in the urine would be consistent with the diagnosis of PIH. This question has a false response stem, so the correct answer is something that the nurse would NOT expect to find in an assessment of the client.

2. CORRECT. In PIH, the nurse would expect to find an increased deep tendon reflex, not a decreased deep tendon reflex.

> **TEST-TAKING TIP:** Because this question has a false response stem, the correct answer is something the nurse would NOT expect to find in an assessment of the client.

3. INCORRECT. This would be consistent with the admitting diagnosis. Manifestations of PIH include proteinuria, edema, and elevated blood pressure. Blood pressure of 148/98 is elevated and would be consistent with the diagnosis of PIH. The correct answer is something the nurse would NOT expect to find in an assessment of the client.

4. INCORRECT. This would be consistent with the admitting diagnosis. Manifestations of PIH include edema, proteinuria, and elevated blood pressure. A finding of 1+ pitting sacral edema would be consistent with the diagnosis of PIH. The correct answer is something the nurse would NOT expect to find in an assessment of the client.

9. When the nurse enters a client's room, the client's son tells the nurse, "You people can't do anything right. Ever since my parent was admitted to this hospital, it has been one mistake after another. I am taking my parent out of here before you kill my parent." The nurse's most helpful response to the son is:

1. "You feel that your parent is not being well cared for?"
2. "We have the best intentions for the clients."
3. "I'll get the supervisor for you."
4. "Your parent hasn't complained about the care. What specifically is the problem?"

1. CORRECT. This response uses the communication tool of restatement and focuses on the issue. This response encourages the son to express his concerns to the nurse. The nurse needs more information from the client before the problem can be solved. This response also focuses on the "here and now."

2. INCORRECT. This response is a defensive remark by the nurse, which is a communication block. This response implies that whatever is bothering the son cannot be valid, and this response may escalate the situation. A therapeutic response would encourage the son to tell the nurse why he feels upset concerning his parent's care.

3. INCORRECT. *The son is the client in this communication question. This response puts the client's feelings on hold by asking him to wait until the supervisor arrives. Therapeutic communication addresses the "here and now," and does not "pass the buck" to another person. Indeed, the supervisor may become involved, but the best response by the nurse is to address the client's immediate needs.*

4. INCORRECT. *The son is the client in this communication question. This response focuses on the parent, but the son is the one who has voiced concerns to the nurse. This response implies that the son's feelings cannot be valid since his parent has not voiced any complaints. This devalues the client's feelings and is not therapeutic.*

10. **After a myocardial infarction, which vital signs assessment should the nurse recognize as possible indications of cardiogenic shock?**

    1. BP - 180/100, P - 90, irregular.
    2. BP - 130/80, P - 100 regular.
    3. BP - 90/50, P - 50 regular.
    4. BP - 80/60, P - 110, irregular.

    1. INCORRECT. *These vital signs are not seen in a shock-like state.*
    2. INCORRECT. *These vital signs are within normal limits. Recall the pathophysiology of shock, and make a more appropriate selection.*
    3. INCORRECT. *This is only partially correct. The client in cardiogenic shock will be hypotensive, but will not be bradycardic.*
    4. **CORRECT. *The classic signs of cardiogenic shock are low blood pressure, rapid and weak pulse, cold, clammy skin, decreased urinary output, and cerebral hypoxia.***

11. **An 18-year-old client is hospitalized for treatment of severe depression. Which nursing approach would be most therapeutic to include in the client's plan of care?**

    1. Giving the client choices.
    2. Spending time with the client.
    3. Providing a chess game.
    4. Encouraging decision-making.

    1. INCORRECT. *This is not an appropriate nursing approach to include in this client's plan of care. Making choices is difficult for a depressed client.*

    TEST-TAKING TIP: Note that this option is very similar to Option 4. Neither one can be correct! Such similar options should be eliminated.

    2. **CORRECT. *Because depressed clients frequently have suicidal tendencies, spending time with the client will provide for safety. Depression also involves diminished self-esteem, and spending time with the client conveys that the client is worth the nurse's time and attention. This action is therapeutic for the client and provides for safety.***

3. INCORRECT. *This is not the most therapeutic approach for this client. An intellectual game such as chess would not be a good activity for a depressed client. Non-intellectual activities such as latch hook or needle work would be a better choice. Read all of the other options, and then try to select the best one.*

4. INCORRECT. *This is not an appropriate nursing approach to include in this client's plan of care. Decision-making is difficult for a depressed client.*

TEST-TAKING TIP: Note that this option is very similar to Option 1. Neither one can be correct! Such similar options should be eliminated.

12. **A two-year-old is hospitalized with bacterial pneumonia. The nurse will monitor the client's respiratory status closely. Which manifestations would the nurse identify as the earliest indication of respiratory difficulty?**

    1. Respiratory rate of 40 to 48.
    2. Blood pressure of 80/60.
    3. Cyanosis of mucous membranes.
    4. Circumoral/periorbital pallor.

    1. **CORRECT. *One early indication of respiratory difficulty is an increased respiratory rate. A respiratory rate of 40 to 48 is rapid for a two-year-old.***
    2. INCORRECT. *A blood pressure of 80/60 is within normal limits for a two-year-old and does not indicate increased respiratory difficulty.*
    3. INCORRECT. *Cyanosis of mucous membranes is certainly a sign of respiratory difficulty, but it is a late sign. The nurse should be alert for early signs so that appropriate intervention can begin.*
    4. INCORRECT. *Circumoral/periorbital pallor is certainly a sign of respiratory difficulty. However, this is a late sign. The nurse should be alert for early signs so that appropriate intervention can begin.*

13. **A client is in labor and is admitted with a blood pressure of 86/52. She is four centimeters dilated and uncomfortable. The nurse should give immediate consideration to which nursing action?**

    1. Call the physician to report the blood pressure.
    2. Turn the client on her side and retake her blood pressure.
    3. Reassure the client that everything is all right.
    4. Ask the client if she would like some pain medication.

    1. INCORRECT. *While it is important to notify the physician, it is not the immediate action by the nurse. The need for adequate blood pressure is a physiological need that requires immediate intervention. Try to identify another option that addresses this need.*
    2. **CORRECT. *Supine hypotension is a frequent cause of low blood pressure in pregnant clients. By turning the client on her side and retaking the blood pressure, the nurse is attempting to correct the low blood pressure and then reassessing. The need for adequate blood pressure is a physiological need that requires immediate intervention.***

3. *INCORRECT. Reassuring the client that everything is all right is not a priority action and may be false reassurance. Maslow's hierarchy of needs indicates that physiological needs should receive priority.*

4. *INCORRECT. The issue in this question is labor and low blood pressure. The need for adequate blood pressure is a physiological need that requires immediate intervention. This option is focused on the client's discomfort, which is not life-threatening and may not require medication once other comfort measures can be instituted. The client's comfort should be addressed as soon as the nurse has determined that the blood pressure is stable.*

14. **During a client's postoperative recovery from an ileostomy, the nurse begins teaching stoma care. The client refuses to look at the ostomy and tells the nurse, "I'd rather be dead than have to live with this all my life." The appropriate nursing response is:**

    1. "I can't imagine what you must be feeling; it must be awful."
    2. "I'll call your physician and see if something can be ordered to help you relax."
    3. "There's no reason to feel like that. Things will get better."
    4. "You appear upset. Would you like to talk?"

    1. *INCORRECT. This response may appear empathetic, but it is excessive and is not therapeutic. Expressing excessive approval can be as harmful to the nurse/client relationship as stating disapproval.*
    2. *INCORRECT. This response ignores the client's statement and changes the subject, which conveys a lack of empathy. This response does not encourage the client to express feelings.*
    3. *INCORRECT. This response offers false reassurance to the client, which is a block to therapeutic communication.*
    4. **CORRECT. This response uses the therapeutic communication tool of empathy, and in a non-threatening manner encourages the client to verbalize negative feelings. It conveys to the client a caring attitude and a willingness to listen.**

15. **A female client was hospitalized for major depression and treated with nortriptyline (Pamelor). As the client is preparing for discharge, which statement by the client would indicate to the nurse the need for further instruction?**

    1. "I'm glad this medicine helps me. My husband and I would like to start our family as soon as possible."
    2. "If I should feel hopeless and suicidal again, I have the telephone number of my therapist to call for help."
    3. "I hope I will not have to continue taking medicine forever. I guess I'll have to see how I do."
    4. "I plan to see my psychiatrist regularly. If I continue to do well, I can probably stop taking my medication in nine to 12 months."

1. **CORRECT. This statement indicates that the client needs further instruction. Tricyclic antidepressants should be avoided during pregnancy, especially during the first trimester, because they are associated with fetal anomalies.**

2. *INCORRECT. This statement by the client does not indicate that the client needs further instruction. Since 60% of depressed persons experience suicidal thoughts, each hospitalized client should have a plan for obtaining help if these thoughts recur after discharge. The client's statement indicates that she has a good plan to follow, which the nurse should reinforce. The stem asks for the statement that indicates a knowledge deficit.*

3. *INCORRECT. This is a realistic statement. It does not indicate a need for further instruction. An estimated 15% of clients with depressive illness develop chronic or recurring manifestations of depression. Clients should remain under the care of a mental health professional after hospital discharge so their condition can be monitored. The stem in this question asks for the statement that indicates a knowledge deficit.*

4. *INCORRECT. This statement by the client is appropriate. Most clients remain on their antidepressant for nine to 12 months after recovering from an episode of depression. A rebound depression can occur if the medication is discontinued too soon. This statement by the client does not indicate a need for further instruction. The stem in this question asks for the statement that indicates a knowledge deficit.*

16. **A client who had foot surgery has just returned from the recovery room. The nurse's initial assessment indicates the client is stable. An hour later, the client's roommate turns on the call light and tells the nurse that the client has gotten up and hopped on one foot to the bathroom, using the IV pole for support. The initial nursing action to provide for the client's safety is to:**

    1. Open the bathroom door to assess if the client is okay.
    2. Assist the client in ambulating back to bed and get the client a bedpan.
    3. Explain to the client that it is not safe to be hopping around on one foot.
    4. Get a wheelchair and help the client back to bed when the client is done in the bathroom.

    1. *INCORRECT. This action is inappropriate. Even though the client should not have hopped to the bathroom, the nurse should respect the client's privacy and knock on the door before going in.*
    2. *INCORRECT. This action is inappropriate and unsafe. The client will have to hop back to bed with the nurse's support, which is not a very stable method of ambulation.*
    3. *INCORRECT. This is not the priority action. Since the client is already in the bathroom, getting the client safely back to bed is the priority issue for the nurse.*
    4. **CORRECT. Since the client is already in the bathroom, allow the client to void and then use a wheelchair to return the client to bed. This is an implementation question, and the stem asks you to prioritize the actions. This option meets the physiological and safety needs of the client, while also respecting the client's privacy.**

17. An elderly client was hospitalized for observation after experiencing a fall when walking for exercise. The client is to ambulate for the first time since the fall, but tells the nurse, "I'm afraid to get up." The best response by the nurse is:

   1. "There is nothing to be afraid of. The order wouldn't have been written if your doctor didn't think that you were ready."
   2. "Tell me what concerns you about getting up today."
   3. "I will have another person here to help you when you get up."
   4. "Are you afraid of falling again?"

   1. *INCORRECT. This is not the best response by the nurse because it does not facilitate a response from the client. It devalues the client's concerns by making the doctor's orders seem more important. It also focuses on the doctor and not on the client. A therapeutic response focuses on the client's feelings.*
   2. **CORRECT. This nursing response focuses on the client's feelings, and it gives value to the client's statement by directly addressing the client's concerns. This response uses the therapeutic communication tool of clarification and encourages the client to express to the nurse any concerns about ambulating.**
   3. *INCORRECT. This response may not address the client's concerns, since the nurse does not know why the client is afraid. Clarification is necessary before the nurse can plan to meet the client's needs. This response focuses on the nurse's action, and not on the client's feelings.*
   4. *INCORRECT. The nurse does not know why the client is afraid, but this is not the best clarification question to ask because it can be answered with a simple "yes" or "no" answer. The nurse should encourage the client to express any feelings.*

18. To safely assess for correct placement of a nasogastric tube, the nurse should:

   1. Instill 30 mL of saline to assess client tolerance.
   2. Instill 10 mL of air into the tube and listen for gurgling sounds with a stethoscope over the gastric area.
   3. Aspirate stomach contents with a syringe.
   4. Place the end of the tube in water to assess for bubbling.

   1. *INCORRECT. This procedure could be dangerous if the tube was incorrectly positioned in the lungs. Select a safer action.*
   2. *INCORRECT. This method does not provide for a sufficient amount of air to reach the stomach and make any gurgling sounds. At least 30 mL of air is needed for this test. There is a safer and more reliable method among the options given.*
   3. **CORRECT. Placement should be checked by aspirating gastric contents with a syringe and testing the pH of the aspirate.**
   4. *INCORRECT. This could be dangerous to the client if the tube was incorrectly positioned in the lungs, because the client could aspirate the water in the glass. Select a safer, more reliable option.*

19. A psychiatric client is re-hospitalized after deciding to discontinue prescribed medication. The client has responded well to the support of the nurse-client relationship. The client's discharge plans include living with the parents and attending a job training program during the day. What is the most important goal for the client's remaining sessions with the nurse?

   1. Reinforce the importance of taking the medications as prescribed.
   2. Anticipate future problems and how the client might handle them.
   3. Terminate the nurse-client relationship.
   4. Promote the client's self-confidence.

   1. *INCORRECT. Reinforcing the client's medication regime is an important component of discharge planning, especially for this client, who had to be re-hospitalized after deciding to discontinue taking medications. However, it is not the most important goal at this time. There is a better option.*
   2. *INCORRECT. This is an important component of discharge planning, but it is not the most important goal at this time.*
   3. **CORRECT. The nurse should focus on ending their relationship by exploring the client's responses to the separation and dealing with any feelings of rejection that the client may have. This is the most important goal at this time, as it greatly affects the client's ability to establish positive relationships with health care providers in the future.**
   4. *INCORRECT. Promoting self-confidence is usually a component of the nursing care plan, but it is not the most important goal at this time.*

20. The nurse knows the discharge teaching for a client with Hepatitis A virus is successful when the client indicates it would be unsafe to:

   1. Donate blood.
   2. Eat fried foods.
   3. Vacation in a foreign country.
   4. Order a salad in a restaurant.

   1. **CORRECT. Once a person has been infected with Hepatitis A virus, that person can never donate blood.**
   2. *INCORRECT. The client should not need to avoid fried foods permanently. Dietary fat is not contraindicated, but it may not be well tolerated. After recovering, the client should be able to tolerate fats within two months.*
   3. *INCORRECT. It is not necessary for the client to refrain from vacationing abroad. This in itself has no direct correlation to Hepatitis A virus.*
   4. *INCORRECT. The client's fear is real if the initial cause of Hepatitis A was from eating at a restaurant. It is not necessary for the client to refrain from eating in restaurants, or from ordering salads, however, since this in itself has no direct correlation to Hepatitis A virus.*

21. **A client is hospitalized following myocardial infarction. When transferring the client from a cart to the bed, the priority nursing action is to:**

    1. Ask the client to place the arms on the chest.
    2. Lock the wheels on the cart and the bed.
    3. Have at least four people help with the transfer.
    4. Use a draw sheet to move the client.

    1. INCORRECT. Although placing the arms across the chest helps protect the arms from injury, this option is not the priority action requested by the stem of the question.

    2. CORRECT. This is the priority action for transferring a client. Locking the wheels prevents the cart or bed from moving apart or away from the client, and thus prevents the client from falling to the floor.

    3. INCORRECT. Four people may or may not be the number needed for a transfer. The number will depend on the size of the client and the size of the persons performing the transfer. The case scenario does not provide enough information to establish this number of staff as necessary for the transfer.

    4. INCORRECT. A draw sheet is often used to transfer clients between two level horizontal surfaces; however, this is neither a requirement nor a priority action.

22. **The nurse understands the inaccurate statement about reality testing is that it is:**

    1. An ego function.
    2. Impaired in psychotic individuals.
    3. Impaired in persons who are mentally retarded.
    4. The capacity to distinguish thoughts, feelings, fantasies, and other experiences that originate inside the individual from those that are part of the outside environment.

    1. INCORRECT. This statement is accurate. Reality testing is an important ego function. Reality testing refers to the capacity to distinguish inner experiences from those that occur in the environment, and the capacity to establish intact ego boundaries. The stem of the question asks you to select an INACCURATE statement about reality testing.

    2. INCORRECT. This statement is accurate. Reality testing is impaired in psychotic individuals. In psychotic disorders, the individual can no longer tell whether personal thoughts and feelings come from within, but instead may experience them as hallucinations and delusions originating from elsewhere. The stem of the question asks you to select an INACCURATE statement about reality testing.

    3. CORRECT. Reality testing is NOT impaired in persons who are mentally retarded, unless they are also psychotic. This is the INACCURATE statement sought in this test question.

    4. INCORRECT. This is an accurate statement about reality testing. It is not the correct option in this question because the stem of the question asks you to select an option that is INACCURATE.

23. **The client is to receive a medication for control of tachycardia and an irregular heart rate. The nurse obtains the following vital signs prior to administering this medication: blood pressure 98/54, pulse 48 bpm., respirations 30, and temperature 98 degrees F. The client's skin is cool, with cyanosis of the fingers and lips. The appropriate nursing action is to:**

    1. Administer the medication as ordered by the physician.
    2. Omit the medication for a day or two, depending on the client's response and manifestations.
    3. Notify the physician concerning the client's status before administering the medication.
    4. Give the client one half of the ordered dose.

    1. INCORRECT. Administering a medication that decreases the heart rate of a client with a pulse of 48 is unsafe, since the pulse rate may decrease even further. A pulse rate of 48 does not fall within the normal range, and results in a physiological need for oxygen for this client.

    2. INCORRECT. A pulse rate of 48 results in a physiological need for oxygen for this client. Withholding the medication is a possible nursing action, since the result of this action may be an increase in pulse rate. However, withholding the medication alone does not address all of the physiological needs identified in the case scenario. Be sure to read all the options before selecting the best one.

    3. CORRECT. The assessment data gathered by the nurse indicates the client is exhibiting manifestations that are not within the normal parameters. A pulse rate of 48 results in a physiological need for oxygen for this client. Withholding the medication until the physician has been notified addresses the immediate physiological need of the client. The information needs to be communicated to the physician, who will determine which medical interventions are necessary.

    4. INCORRECT. Changing or altering an ordered medication is a medical intervention, not a nursing action.

24. **The nurse is preparing a teaching plan for a client being discharged following major abdominal surgery. The client will be doing personal dressing changes at home. Which technique is the most important for the nurse to include in the discharge teaching plan?**

    1. Opening bandages properly to maintain their sterility.
    2. Maintaining strict aseptic technique.
    3. Proper gloving technique.
    4. Good handwashing technique.

    1. INCORRECT. The client is at risk for the transmission of microorganisms that may cause infection. The nurse should instruct the client in the proper method of opening bandages and other measures to prevent infection while changing the dressing. The home environment does not lend itself to the practice of aseptic technique, however, so the nurse must help the client improvise with the resources available. What is the most important action in preventing the spread of infection?

2. *INCORRECT. The client is at risk for the transmission of microorganisms that may cause an infection. The home environment does not lend itself to the practice of aseptic technique, however, so the nurse must help the client improvise with the resources available. What is the most important action in preventing the spread of infection?*

3. *INCORRECT. The client is at risk for the transmission of microorganisms that may cause an infection. The home environment does not lend itself to the practice of aseptic technique, however, so the nurse must help the client improvise with the resources available. What is the most important action in preventing the spread of infection?*

4. **CORRECT. The client is at risk for the transmission of microorganisms that may cause an infection. The home environment may not lend itself to the entire practice of aseptic technique, so the nurse must help the client improvise with the resources available. Handwashing is the most important and most basic technique in preventing and controlling the transmission of pathogens and it should be practiced in every case.**

25. **A premature infant weighed only three pounds and seven ounces at birth. Following a lengthy stay in the hospital, the infant's weight has increased to five pounds so the infant will be discharged soon. Which statement by the mother would indicate to the nurse that additional teaching is needed?**

    1. "My baby is so fragile that I will need to be extra careful with everything I do for the baby."
    2. "I know that my baby will need to see the doctor regularly for awhile, and I have the appointments on my calendar."
    3. "My mother is going to stay with me for several weeks to help me with my older children."
    4. "I have the nursery, clothing, bottles, and diapers all ready for the day we bring our baby home."

    1. **CORRECT. Caring for a premature infant at home should not be any different from caring for a full-term baby. This statement does reflect a need for further instruction.**
    2. *INCORRECT. This statement by the client is appropriate and does not reflect a need for more instruction. Regular doctor appointments are especially important for premature infants because there is a greater risk for anemia and failure to thrive. You are looking for a statement by the mother that indicates a knowledge deficit.*
    3. *INCORRECT. Extra help with household chores and older children is beneficial support when mother and baby are adjusting to a new schedule. This statement by the client is appropriate. You are looking for a statement by the mother that indicates a knowledge deficit.*
    4. *INCORRECT. This comment indicates that the mother is prepared to provide care for the baby at home. You are looking for a statement by the mother that indicates a knowledge deficit.*

26. **The doctor finds a lump in the client's breast and says that a biopsy needs to be done. The client asks the nurse, "Do you think it is cancer?" The initial nursing response should be:**

    1. "You seem to be worried about what the doctor may find."
    2. "Do you have a family history of breast cancer?"
    3. "We won't know anything until the biopsy is done."
    4. "Most lumps are not cancerous, so you really shouldn't worry."

    1. **CORRECT. This is a good therapeutic response. Communication theory states that the nurse should focus on the client's feelings. This response focuses on the client's concerns that she may have cancer. This response addresses the "here and now," using the therapeutic communication tools of empathy and clarification.**
    2. *INCORRECT. This should not be the initial response by the nurse because it is not therapeutic for this worried client. The response focuses on the client's family history, not on the client's feelings. The stem of the question asks what should be the initial response. After the client's feelings are addressed, then information may be obtained concerning the client's family history of breast cancer.*
    3. *INCORRECT. This response is not therapeutic. The response does not answer the client's question or promote further expression of the client's feelings. It blocks communication by putting the client's feelings of fear on hold.*
    4. *INCORRECT. This response is not therapeutic. The response offers false assurance and does not encourage the client to express her feelings about cancer. Telling the client not to worry devalues the client's feelings.*

27. **A client has just been diagnosed with advanced, untreatable cancer. When the nurse enters the room to set up the bath equipment, the client says, "I'm not an invalid, you know. I can take care of myself. Get out and leave me alone." What is the best nursing response?**

    1. "I know that you are not an invalid. I was just trying to help you."
    2. "It sounds to me like you are angry about something. Did somebody do something wrong?"
    3. "You are pretty upset. Let's talk about it."
    4. "I'll just set up this equipment for you to bathe and come back later when you're not so angry."

    1. *INCORRECT. This is an inappropriate response because it focuses on the nurse and not on the client.*
    2. *INCORRECT. This response incorrectly assumes the client is angry, and it focuses on inappropriate persons and issues. When the nurse asks if "somebody" did something wrong, the focus is on "somebody" else rather than on the client's feelings.*
    3. **CORRECT. This is the best response because it addresses the emotional state of the client. By stating that the client is upset, the nurse uses the communication tool of clarification. Clarification is used to promote therapeutic communication, which focuses first on the client's feelings.**

4. *INCORRECT. This option does not promote any communication with the client. It implies that the client's behavior is inappropriate and that the nurse is not willing to deal with it.*

28. A six-year-old child is admitted with a spiral fracture of the humerus and multiple bruises of the forearm. The physician states that the injuries and other signs are suspicious for abuse. The nurse's initial goal is to:

1. Prevent further abuse of the client.
2. Encourage the client to express any feelings.
3. Determine who is responsible for the abuse.
4. Teach the parents the appropriate methods of discipline.

1. ***CORRECT. This is the nurse's initial goal because the immediate safety of the child is the priority. After the child's safety has been ensured, then interventions to decrease the chances of further abuse (such as education of parents) can be implemented.***

2. *INCORRECT. This is not the nurse's initial goal. While encouraging the child to express feelings is important, it is not the most important nursing responsibility at this time.*

TEST-TAKING TIP: Use Maslow's hierarchy of needs to prioritize the nurse's actions.

3. *INCORRECT. This is not the nurse's main responsibility. There is a more important nursing responsibility at this time. TEST-TAKING TIP: Use Maslow's hierarchy of needs to prioritize the nurse's actions.*

4. *INCORRECT. This is not the nurse's initial goal. While it is important to eventually teach the parents appropriate methods of discipline, it is not the most important nursing responsibility at this time. TEST-TAKING TIP: Use Maslow's hierarchy of needs to prioritize the nurse's actions.*

29. While caring for a client, the nurse should practice good body mechanics to reduce the chance of muscle strain. In using good body mechanics, the nurse would avoid:

1. Moving muscles quickly, using short tugs.
2. Using the longest and strongest muscles of the body.
3. Leaning toward objects being pushed.
4. Carrying objects close to the body .

1. ***CORRECT. This action is incorrect and should be avoided. Jerky movements produce increased strain on muscles and are usually uncomfortable for the client.***

2. *INCORRECT. This action uses good body mechanics because the longest, strongest muscles are less likely to become injured than the small muscles. The question asks you to identify something the nurse would AVOID doing.*

3. *INCORRECT. This is a correct action, using good body mechanics. Body weight adds force to muscle action when pushing any object. The question asks you to identify something the nurse would AVOID doing.*

4. *INCORRECT. Carrying objects close to the body (without touching your clothing) uses good body mechanics. When objects are close to the body, the line of gravity is within the body's base of support which improves balance and reduces strain on the arm muscles. The question asks you to identify something the nurse would AVOID doing.*

30. An elderly client is admitted to the hospital with pneumonia. The client's daughter, who takes care of the client at home, tells the nurse, "I'm so glad my parent is here. You can provide much better care than I can." The best nursing response to the daughter is:

1. "We do have the equipment and people to take care of sick clients."
2. "It is not easy to care for the elderly. How do you manage?"
3. "Your daughter takes good care of you at home, doesn't she?"
4. "Are you feeling guilty because your parent has pneumonia?"

1. *INCORRECT. This is not the best response by the nurse because it does not focus on the appropriate person. Because the daughter has expressed her feelings to the nurse, she is the client in this case scenario. This response also focuses on inappropriate issues concerning other people and hospital equipment. To be therapeutic, the nurse's response should focus on the daughter's feelings and concerns.*

2. ***CORRECT. This response uses the communication tool of showing empathy, and asks for clarification of the statement made to the nurse.***

TEST-TAKING TIP: Be sure to correctly identify the client in communication questions. The daughter is the client in this question, and the nurse's response should address her concerns. Note that Options 1 & 3 focus on inappropriate issues, and Option 4 implies to the client that may be to blame for her parent's pneumonia.

3. *INCORRECT. This response is inappropriate because it is not directed towards the appropriate person. The parent is the person with the medical problem, but the daughter is the client in this test question. The daughter expressed her feelings to the nurse so the nurse's response should be addressed to her.*

4. *INCORRECT. This response is inappropriate because it may appear to place blame on the daughter for her parent's pneumonia. This type of response can put the client on the defensive, which is not therapeutic. Remember, the daughter is the client in this question.*

31. A client has pregnancy-induced hypertension (PIH). In planning care for this client prior to delivery, the most essential nursing order is to:

1. Assess fluid balance hourly and maintain optimum placental perfusion.
2. Monitor urine output and assure a brief rest period every shift.
3. Check the blood pressure before and after each time the client is out of bed.
4. Observe for amount of edema and provide for diversionary activities.

1. **CORRECT. Fluid balance has a relationship to blood pressure and should be assessed frequently. Assessment of fluid balance should include recording of intake and output, measurement of blood pressure, and observation of amount of edema. To maintain optimum placental perfusion, the nurse should assist the client to turn from side to side, but remain in a lateral position. This is the most essential nursing order for this client's plan of care. This question uses the planning phase of the nursing process.**
2. *INCORRECT. Monitoring urine output is an important assessment because oliguria could indicate renal damage in a client with PIH, but output should be monitored more frequently than once a shift. Also, the client should be on bed rest to decrease the need for oxygen by the cells, which will decrease cardiac workload. A brief rest period every shift is not adequate.*
3. *INCORRECT. It is true that the blood pressure should be monitored frequently; if the blood pressure is too high, drugs may be used to control it. However, the client should not be getting out of bed for activities because bed rest is necessary to decrease the cell's need for oxygen, which will decrease cardiac workload.*
4. *INCORRECT. The nurse should observe for the amount of edema and should provide diversionary activities for the client. This is not, however, the most essential nursing order for this client.*

32. A client sustained a T-4 spinal cord injury. While doing morning assessments four weeks post-injury, the nurse discovers the client's BP is 280/140 and the client is complaining of nasal stuffiness and a severe, pounding headache. The first nursing action is to:

1. Sit the client upright.
2. Call the physician.
3. Check the client's bladder for distension.
4. Administer the prescribed antihypertensive.

1. **CORRECT. Since autonomic hyperreflexia is a medical emergency, the first action is to lower the BP. By sitting the client upright, compensatory orthostatic hypotension is used to lower the BP.**
2. *INCORRECT. This is important but it is not the first nursing action. Calling the physician is important after nursing measures have been initiated to lower the BP. What should the nurse do first?*

3. *INCORRECT. This should be done to assess the cause of hyperreflexia, but the first goal is to lower the BP and, ultimately, to prevent stroke. What should the nurse do first?*
4. *INCORRECT. This is not the first action because causing orthostatic hypotension will provide the same results initially. Antihypertensives are used only if non-pharmacologic methods are unsuccessful. What should the nurse do first?*

33. A client is in the hospital with renal failure and is on fluid restriction. The nurse would avoid:

1. Furnishing a variety of fluids in small containers.
2. Informing the client and family about the restriction.
3. Allowing the client to help keep a record of oral intake.
4. Providing fluids only during meal times.

1. *INCORRECT. This is an appropriate nursing measure that allows for choices and variety. Look for something the nurse should NOT do.*
2. *INCORRECT. Informing the client and the family of the restriction is an appropriate nursing action that will make compliance with the restriction more likely. The stem of the question is asking for something the nurse should NOT do.*
3. *INCORRECT. This is an appropriate nursing action that promotes participation of the client in her own care. The stem of the question is asking for something the nurse should NOT do.*
4. **CORRECT. This is the inappropriate action. Since the client may become thirsty at times other than meal times, this nursing measure can lead to noncompliance on the part of the client and family.**

34. The physician has ordered a client to be discharged on a 2,000 calorie-per-day diet. What is the most important nursing action in developing a teaching plan for this client's diet?

1. Obtain sample menus from the dietitian to give to the client.
2. Ask the client to identify the types of foods usually eaten and preferred.
3. Tell the client that all of the client's previous eating habits will have to be changed.
4. Advise the client to buy only dietetic foods.

1. *INCORRECT. Sample menus may be helpful in providing the client with ideas for new foods or exchanges. However, this is not the most important nursing action in developing a diet teaching plan for this client.*
2. **CORRECT. Asking what types of foods the client prefers provides an opportunity for the nurse to include these foods in the client's diet. This will help promote the client's compliance.**
3. *INCORRECT. The client may have to change some eating habits, but not ALL of them. Also, telling the client what to do is inappropriate. This option also fails to give the client any useful information to use in complying.*

TEST-TAKING TIP: Note that the absolute word "all" in this option is a clue that this is probably an incorrect option.

4. *INCORRECT. This option is incorrect because fresh fruits, vegetables, and many other unprepared foods are permitted in a diabetic diet, and the diabetic may also use some prepared foods that are not labeled "dietetic." This option is also incorrect because there are not enough dietetic foods available to meet all of the client's dietary requirements.*

35. **An eight-year-old client is admitted to the hospital with a diagnosis of acute rheumatic fever. Immediately after admission, which nursing assessment is most important?**

   1. Auscultation of the rate and characteristics of heart sounds.
   2. Determining the location and severity of joint pain.
   3. Identifying the degree of anxiety related to the diagnosis.
   4. Determining the family's emotional and financial needs.

   1. ***CORRECT. This is the priority assessment because tachycardia and cardiac murmur indicate cardiac involvement, which may lead to serious and life-threatening complications.***
   2. *INCORRECT. Pain in one or more joints is characteristic of rheumatic fever and would be of concern to the nurse. However, because joint pain is not life-threatening and since there are usually no permanent sequelae, this is not the priority assessment.*
   3. *INCORRECT. Anxiety related to the diagnosis of rheumatic fever and the manifestations and treatment of rheumatic fever is expected and would be of concern to the nurse. This anxiety is not life-threatening, however, and would not receive top priority during the initial assessment.*
   4. *INCORRECT. The family's emotional needs at this time are of concern to the nurse. The length and cost of the treatment needed for rheumatic fever may place a burden on the family's emotional and financial resources. However, this would not be the top priority during the initial assessment of the child.*

36. **A client recently diagnosed with multiple sclerosis questions the nurse concerning the usual course of the disease. What would be the most appropriate response by the nurse?**

   1. "Each client is different. We cannot tell what will happen."
   2. "I can see that you are worried, but it's too soon to predict what will happen."
   3. "Usually, acute episodes are followed by remissions, which may last a long time."
   4. "It's too early to think about the future; let's focus on the present and go day-by-day."

1. *INCORRECT. This is not an appropriate response because it provides the client with no information and blocks further communication..*
2. *INCORRECT. Although the nurse acknowledges the client's feelings with this response, the nurse then blocks communication by not providing any information to help address the client's fears.*
3. ***CORRECT. This is the most appropriate response because the nurse provides factual information while giving the client some realistic hope.***
4. *INCORRECT. This is not an appropriate response because giving advice is a block to communication and will stop the client from feeling free to express concerns and fears.*

37. **While transferring a client with left-leg weakness from the bed to a wheelchair, the priority nursing action is to:**

   1. Have the seat of the wheelchair at a right angle to the bed.
   2. Lock the wheels on the bed and the wheelchair.
   3. Allow the client to do as much as possible to increase sense of independence.
   4. Tell the client to lock the hands around the nurse's neck to provide a sense of security.

   1. *INCORRECT. This is an unsafe nursing action. This position would require the client to pivot 180 degrees to get into the seat of the wheelchair. The seat of the wheelchair should be parallel with and close to the bed to allow easy access for the client.*
   2. ***CORRECT. Locking the wheels of both bed and wheelchair provides for the client's safety by not allowing the equipment to move away from the client, thereby risking an injury from a fall.***

TEST-TAKING TIP: Maslow's hierarchy of needs indicates that when there is no immediate physiological need, safety needs receive priority.

   3. *INCORRECT. Although encouraging independence is important, the client's safety is the most important consideration. A client with a weakened lower extremity is at risk for falling.*
   4. *INCORRECT. This action is unsafe. The client can place the hands on the shoulders of the nurse, but not around the nurse's neck. If the client slips, all of client's weight will be placed on the cervical vertebrae of the nurse, which could cause a spinal cord injury.*

38. **A nurse enters the room and finds the parent of a child diagnosed with leukemia crying. The child is currently receiving chemotherapy. The parent says, "I just can't believe my child is going to lose all that beautiful blonde hair!" Which response by the nurse is most therapeutic?**

   1. "Sometimes the hair only thins."
   2. "You're feeling a lot of loss right now."
   3. "Remember, hair loss means the chemotherapy is working!"
   4. "Kids love to wear the special baseball caps we have."

1. *INCORRECT. While this statement may be true, it is not the most therapeutic for the parent at this time. This response minimizes the parent's concerns and feelings and may discourage further communication.*

2. **CORRECT. This is the most therapeutic response by the nurse. This empathetic statement validates the parent's feelings and encourages further communication.**

3. *INCORRECT. This response contains inaccurate information and fails to address the client's feelings. Hair loss occurs because chemotherapy destroys rapidly growing cells, which include hair, linings of the GI tract, and cancer cells. It is not an indication of the effectiveness of the chemotherapy. This response is not therapeutic for the parent.*

4. *INCORRECT. This response is not therapeutic because it does not address the parent's feelings and concerns. It is also not helpful to generalize for all children.*

39. **A client says to the nurse, "I am so frustrated with having five kids. My husband won't do anything to help keep me from getting pregnant." The initial nursing action is to:**

1. Refer the client and spouse to family planning services.
2. Find out if the client could use a contraceptive that would not involve her husband.
3. Inquire what the client means by "being frustrated."
4. Ask the client if her husband is interested in birth control.

1. *INCORRECT. Referring the client to family planning services might be an option, but it is not the first action the nurse should take. The client has already stated that her husband is not interested in birth control measures that involve him.*

2. **CORRECT. Before planning anything, the nurse needs to get more information. Assessment is the first step of the nursing process.**

3. *INCORRECT. Although this response might appear to be a good choice because it uses clarification, the client has already stated that her frustration is due to the number of children. The nurse does not need to assess any more about the client's feelings of frustration.*

4. *INCORRECT. This is incorrect because the client has already stated that her husband is not interested in birth control measures that directly involve him.*

40. **An adult client is diagnosed with pneumonia and is being treated with penicillin G sodium 3 million units IV every four hours. When completing the drug history, it is especially important for the nurse to assess the client for allergies to:**

1. Antituberculars.
2. Calcium channel blockers.
3. Aminoglycosides.
4. Cephalosporins.

1. *INCORRECT. There is no known cross-sensitivity between penicillin and antitubercular medications.*

2. *INCORRECT. There is no known cross-sensitivity between penicillin and calcium channel blockers.*

3. *INCORRECT. There is no known cross-sensitivity between penicillin and aminoglycosides, which is another group of antibiotics.*

4. **CORRECT. The issue in this question is cross-sensitivity. Many clients who are allergic to penicillins are also allergic to cephalosporins, and vice versa. There is a significant risk of cross-sensitivity.**

41. **A client is gravida 5 para 4. During admission, the nurse assesses that contractions are occurring every two minutes and are lasting approximately 45 seconds. The client sayshas been in labor for approximately 10 hours. The priority assessment the nurse needs to make at this time is:**

1. Time the client last ate.
2. Cervical dilatation.
3. Allergies to medications.
4. Vital signs.

1. *INCORRECT. The time the client last ate is not the priority assessment for this client. What is the issue in this question?*

2. **CORRECT. Based upon the stages of labor, full dilation usually takes approximately eight hours in a multi-gravida woman. Since this woman has already been in labor for 10 hours, the nurse's first priority is to assess cervical dilatation to best plan for a safe delivery.**

3. *INCORRECT. This is not the first priority. What is the issue in this question?*

4. *INCORRECT. Although vital signs are important to assess in the mother and the fetus, ifdelivers while you are taking them, the conditions for delivery may not be safe. What is the issue in this question?*

42. **A client is admitted to the hospital at 38 weeks gestation with a large amount of bright red vaginal bleeding. A diagnosis of partial abruptio placenta is made.is on the fetal monitor, and her vital signs are: FH 138 regular, BP 98/52, pulse 118, respirations 24, temperature 97.6 degrees F. Assuming all of the following are ordered by the physician, the nurse should give first priority to which nursing action?**

1. Abdominal-perineal prep.
2. Insert Foley catheter.
3. Sign informed consent for surgery.
4. Start an IV.

1. *INCORRECT. An abdominal prep can be delayed until just prior to the cesarean delivery if it is needed.*

2. *INCORRECT. The Foley catheter can be inserted in the delivery room just prior to the delivery, if it is needed.*

3. *INCORRECT. The consent form, if not signed immediately by the client, can be signed by a family member if the situation warrants. This is not the nurse's priority at this time.*

4. **CORRECT. Insertion of the IV line into this client is the first priority. She is at high risk for shock and if that occurs, it will be very difficult to insert an IV catheter.**

43. **A 15-year-old female client is being seen in the family planning clinic. She says to the nurse that she is nervous and has never had a pelvic examination before. The appropriate response by the nurse is:**

    1. "All you have to do is relax."
    2. "It is only slightly uncomfortable."
    3. "What part of the exam makes you nervous?"
    4. "If you want birth control pills, then a pelvic exam is required."

    1. *INCORRECT. This statement is trite, does not address the client's concerns, and blocks communication by using false reassurance. This response is not therapeutic.*

    2. *INCORRECT. This response does not address the client's concerns and does not encourage further discussion. The response is not therapeutic.*

    3. **CORRECT. This therapeutic response recognizes the client's feelings. It also uses the tool of clarification to encourage the client to tell the nurse more about her concerns.**

    4. *INCORRECT. This statement is true in its literal sense, but the nurse does not know if the client wants birth control pills. Do not "read into" the question. More importantly, however, the client might interpret this statement as expressing disapproval by the nurse. It is non-therapeutic for the nurse to express approval or disapproval. This response also fails to address the feelings that the client has shared with the nurse.*

44. **If a nurse discovered a fire in a client's room, the first nursing action would be to:**

    1. Pull the fire alarm and notify the hospital operator.
    2. Close fire doors and client room doors.
    3. Remove the client from the room.
    4. Place moist towels or blankets at the threshold of the door of the room with the fire.

    1. *INCORRECT. Although pulling the fire alarm and alerting the hospital operator notifies the appropriate individuals who are needed to fight a fire, this is not the first nursing action. The immediate safety of the client in the room with the fire takes priority.*

    2. *INCORRECT. Closing fire doors helps prevent the spread of a fire to other areas of the hospital and closing the clients' room doors helps prevent smoke and fumes from entering their rooms. While this is an important intervention to help protect the other hospitalized clients, there is another action that should be implemented first. The immediate safety of the client in the room with the fire takes priority.*

3. **CORRECT. Moving this client to safety receives first priority. The client in the room with the fire is at highest risk for injury. The smoke from a fire can deprive a client of adequate oxygenation, and the fire poses a direct threat to the safety of this client.**

4. *INCORRECT. Although placing moist towels or blankets at the threshold of the door where the smoke is coming from helps prevent the smoke and fumes from entering other areas, this is an inappropriate action to take at this time. The client in the room with the fire is at risk for injury and oxygen deprivation.*

45. **In assessing an adult client with diabetes mellitus, the nurse identifies an unexpected finding as:**

    1. Possible increased body weight.
    2. Increased urinary output.
    3. Periods of polydypsia.
    4. Altered heart rate and rhythm.

    1. *INCORRECT. An adult diabetic may gain weight, so the word "possible" makes this a true statement. This question has a false response stem, so you are looking for a finding that is UNEXPECTED with this diagnosis.*

    2. *INCORRECT. Increased urinary output is a manifestation of adult diabetes. This question has a false response stem, so you are looking for a finding that is UNEXPECTED with this diagnosis.*

    3. *INCORRECT. Polydipsia is consistent with the diagnosis of adult diabetes. This question has a false response stem, so you are looking for a finding that is UNEXPECTED with this diagnosis.*

    4. **CORRECT. The question has a false response stem, so the answer is something that the nurse would find in an adult diabetic. Altered heart rate and rhythm are NOT characteristic of diabetes. The other three options are distractors: they list manifestations consistent with the diagnosis of adult diabetes mellitus.**

46. **A client, who is paralyzed from the waist down, is to be up in a chair three times a day. What is the best nursing approach when transferring the client from a bed into a wheelchair?**

    1. Place the wheelchair close to the foot of the bed.
    2. Utilize the principles of body mechanics while providing a safe transfer for the client.
    3. Slide the client to the edge of the bed, keeping the nurse's back straight, and use a rocking motion to pull the client.
    4. Place the nurse's arms under the client's axillae from the back of the client.

    1. *INCORRECT. This is an inappropriate action. The wheelchair should be placed as close to the position of the client's buttocks as possible for a safe and easy transfer. The wheelchair should not be placed at the foot of the bed.*

    2. *CORRECT. The nurse is in control of the nurse's own*

body and the client's movement during the transfer. Providing for the safety of the client and utilizing the principles of body mechanics is the best nursing approach.

TEST-TAKING TIP: Options 3 and 4 describe specific actions that are correct in transferring a client, but Option 2 is the best option because it is a more comprehensive or global statement. When more than one option appears correct, look for a global response option.

3. *INCORRECT. This is an appropriate nursing action that addresses the safety of the nurse and client, but it is not the best option. Positioning the client near the edge of the bed reduces the energy required to move the client to the wheelchair, and using leg and arm muscles to move the client protects the nurse's back. However, there is another option that better describes the "best nursing approach" in transferring this client.*

4. *INCORRECT. Supporting the upper portion of the client's body helps to place the weight of the client over the nurse's center of gravity; however, this option is not the best option. Even though this is a correct action that helps provide for the nurse's and the client's safety, there is another option that better describes the "best nursing approach" in transferring this client.*

47. **A client puts the call light on and indicates a need to urinate. The client has had a Foley catheter in place since surgery two days ago. The nurse's initial action is to:**

1. Remind the client that because a Foley catheter is in place, the client does not need to go to the bathroom.
2. Replace the Foley catheter with a new catheter.
3. Explain to the client that the urge to void is a common occurrence for clients who have urinary catheters.
4. Check the catheter and tubing for kinks and note the urine output in the drainage bag.

1. *INCORRECT. This action by the nurse does not meet the client's needs. Although a Foley catheter is in place, it may not be patent. This can result in distention of the bladder and cause the client to feel the urge to void.*

2. *INCORRECT. While a new catheter might be necessary to meet the client's needs, the nurse must first assess the situation further to determine the cause of the client's urge to void. TEST-TAKING TIP: This question is asking for the initial nursing action. Remember the nursing process—assess first.*

3. *INCORRECT. This action is inappropriate because the urge to void usually occurs upon initial insertion of the Foley catheter, not two days afterwards. There are several possible reasons for the client having urgency, and the nurse must attempt to discover the cause in order to meet the client's needs.*

4. **CORRECT. Checking the equipment is the best nursing action, since data will be obtained that will assist the nurse with problem solving.**

TEST-TAKING TIP: This prioritizing question uses the nursing process. The nurse should always assess before planning or implementing a nursing intervention. The nurse does not know the reason for the client's need to void, which means that the implementation actions in Options 1, 2, and 3 cannot be the answer.

48. **A 49-year-old client has been diagnosed with iron deficiency anemia. When teaching the client about diet, the nurse should recommend an increased intake of:**

1. Fresh fruits.
2. Milk and cheese.
3. Organ meats.
4. Whole grain breads.

1. *INCORRECT. This client is deficient in iron. Fruits are a good source of vitamins A and C, not iron. This option does not correctly address the issue in the question.*

2. *INCORRECT. This client is deficient in iron. Dairy products are good sources of high quality complete protein, not iron. This option does not correctly address the issue in the question.*

3. **CORRECT. A diet rich in organ meats provides iron, which is what the client needs to improve the anemia.**

4. *INCORRECT. This client is deficient in iron. Whole grain breads are rich in carbohydrates and dietary fiber, not iron. This option does not correctly address the issue in the question.*

49. **A client is to have a nasogastric tube inserted because of a bowel obstruction. The nurse explains the procedure and is about to begin the insertion when the client says, "No way! You are not putting that hose down my throat. Get away from me." The best nursing response is:**

1. "You have the right to refuse treatment. Why don't you talk to your doctor about it?"
2. "Something is upsetting you. Can you tell me what it is?"
3. "What exactly do you feel about this 'hose'?"
4. "It'll be easier for you to just get it over with. It only gets harder if you get worked up over it and you won't get better without this tube."

1. *INCORRECT. This response puts the client's feelings on hold, referring them to another person at a later time. Although the client has the right to refuse treatment, the nurse should offer an opportunity to express any concerns. This response blocks communication.*

2. **CORRECT. This response addresses the client's feelings. This option uses the communication tool of clarification, which helps the nurse assess the situation. It is more global than Option 3, which focuses only on the client's feelings about the nasogastric tube.**

3. *INCORRECT. This option asks for a response from the client concerning the hose. The nurse does not need information concerning the hose. The nurse needs information concerning the client's feelings about the whole situation.*

4. INCORRECT. This is not the best response because the nurse is blocking communication by giving advice.

50. The nurse tells a client that the doctor has ordered an intravenous line to be started. The client appears to be upset, but says nothing to the nurse. Which is the best nursing response to this situation?

1. "Do you have any questions about the procedure?"
2. "The doctor wants you to have antibiotics, and this method eliminates getting frequent injections."
3. "What is there about this procedure that concerns you?"
4. "It only hurts a little bit. It'll be over before you know it."

1. INCORRECT. This is not the best response because it focuses too narrowly on the procedure. What is the issue in this communication question?

2. INCORRECT. This is an inappropriate response because it focuses on an inappropriate person (the doctor) and raises an inappropriate issue (antibiotics by injection). This response does not promote therapeutic communication.

3. CORRECT. This response uses the communication tool of clarification and invites the client to express concerns and feelings with the nurse.

4. INCORRECT. This option is incorrect. An intravenous puncture hurts more than a little bit. This communication block is identified as false assurance. In this response the nurse is assuming that the client's silence stems from a concern about pain. Which option uses the communication tool of clarification and focuses on the client's feelings?

51. A client shows the nurse the result of a recent tuberculin skin test. The site is red and swollen. The nurse interprets this as the:

1. Client has active tuberculosis.
2. Client has a history of tuberculosis.
3. Tubercle bacillus is in the active pulmonary stage of tuberculosis.
4. Client has had contact with the tubercle bacillus.

1. INCORRECT. A skin test that shows a marked change indicates only that the client was exposed to the tubercle bacillus. A positive chest x-ray and a positive sputum culture for the acid-fast bacillus would indicate active tuberculosis.

> **TEST-TAKING TIP:** Note that Options 1 and 3 are very similar. Two options that use the same idea must be distractors and can be eliminated.

2. INCORRECT. A positive tuberculin skin test means only that the client has been exposed to the tubercle bacillus. This does not indicate that the client has had tuberculosis.

3. INCORRECT. A positive skin test does not indicate an active lesion. Further tests are necessary to diagnose active tuberculosis.

4. CORRECT. A marked reaction to the skin test only indicates exposure to the tubercle bacillus. This question requires an understanding of what a positive reaction to the tuberculin skin test indicates.

52. A client is in the hospital and has weakness on the left side because of a stroke. The client becomes upset when eating because liquids drool out of the weak side of the mouth. What nursing intervention would be most appropriate?

1. Providing only pureed and solid foods to prevent drooling.
2. Letting a member of the family assist with the client's feedings.
3. Teaching the client how to drink fluids on the unaffected side to prevent drooling.
4. Having the client use a syringe to squirt liquids into the back of the mouth.

1. INCORRECT. Eliminating liquids from the client's diet is inappropriate, since fluids are a basic physiological need.

2. INCORRECT. This is not the most appropriate nursing intervention. This option does not solve the problem of the drooling fluids and does not promote independence in this client.

3. CORRECT. This is the most appropriate nursing intervention because it promotes independence and addresses the problem of drooling, which is the issue in this question. The client still has control over swallowing and tongue motion on the unaffected side.

4. INCORRECT. This is not the most appropriate nursing intervention. Although this may help eliminate some drooling, it does not promote normalcy during eating, which can result in a decrease in self-esteem.

53. A 10-year-old client is in sickle cell crisis. Which nursing action is contraindicated?

1. Administer oxygen via nasal cannula as prescribed.
2. Encourage the client to increase oral fluid intake.
3. Administer narcotics only for very severe pain.
4. Encourage as much exercise as possible during the crisis.

1. INCORRECT. This action is appropriate. Hemoglobin S forms a sickled shape in the presence of low oxygen tension, and oxygen is administered to prevent the condition of low oxygen tension. The question is asking you to identify something the nurse should NOT do.

2. INCORRECT. This action is appropriate. High fluid intake prevents dehydration, which would encourage aggregation of the cells and microvascular occlusion. The question is asking you to identify something the nurse should NOT do.

3. *INCORRECT. This action is appropriate. Relief of pain is an important goal during a sickle cell crisis, but physical measures, such as application of heat, should be used whenever they are effective. If physical measures are not effective, non-narcotic analgesics should be tried. Narcotics are administered only for severe pain that is not relieved by physical measures and non-narcotic analgesics. Clients with sickle cell anemia are likely to have pain over an extended period of time, and addiction may become a problem. The question is asking you to identify something the nurse should NOT do.*

4. **CORRECT. This action is inappropriate; the nurse should not encourage exercise. During a sickle cell crisis, exercise should be kept to a minimum. Clients are usually placed on bedrest to decrease the need for oxygen by the cells.**

> **TEST-TAKING TIP:** Note that the word "crisis" appears in the stem of the question and in this option. If you did not know the answer, this is a clue that this option might be correct. However, be sure to always "go with what you know" because that is always the best test-taking strategy.

54. **A client has sustained a basal skull fracture and the nurse notices drainage from the client's right nostril. The priority nursing action is to:**

1. Notify the physician.
2. Suction the nostril.
3. Test the drainage for glucose.
4. Ask the client to blow the nose.

1. *INCORRECT. The nurse has not determined the source of the bleeding and does not have the information that the physician will require. This is a prioritizing question. What should the nurse do first?*

2. *INCORRECT. This action is contraindicated if the drainage is cerebral spinal fluid.*

3. **CORRECT. This is the priority nursing action. Positive glucose on a reagent strip signifies that the drainage is cerebral spinal fluid. This must then be reported to the physician.**

4. *INCORRECT. This action is contraindicated because it may prolong closure of a dural tear and increase the risk of infection.*

55. **If verapamil hydrochloride (Calan) is administered with propranolol (Inderal), the nurse should monitor the client closely for signs of:**

1. Hypertension.
2. Increased peripheral resistance.
3. Bradycardia and heart failure.
4. Diarrhea.

1. *INCORRECT. The client should be monitored for hypotension, not hypertension. Hypotension occurs as both drugs decrease myocardial contractions and lower peripheral resistance.*

2. *INCORRECT. Increased peripheral resistance is the same concept as hypertension. The client should be monitored for hypotension, not hypertension. Hypotension occurs as both drugs decrease myocardial contractions and lower peripheral resistance.*

> **TEST-TAKING TIP:** When two options are similar, such as options 1 and 2, neither can be the correct answer.

3. **CORRECT. Bradycardia and heart failure can occur when these drugs are used together.**

4. *INCORRECT. Nausea and constipation are reported, but not diarrhea.*

56. **In assessing a client after a bronchoscopy, the nurse would give immediate attention to:**

1. Blood-tinged mucous.
2. Complaints of hoarseness when speaking.
3. Irritation and discomfort when swallowing.
4. Difficulty breathing.

1. *INCORRECT. This would not require immediate attention by the nurse. Blood-tinged mucous and sputum are normal after this procedure. The bronchoscope may cause trauma to the tissue of the larynx, trachea, or bronchi when inserted.*

2. *INCORRECT. This complaint is normal after this procedure and would not require the nurse's immediate attention. The client may complain of hoarseness after the bronchoscopy because of the trauma to tissue of the larynx and the trachea.*

3. *INCORRECT. This would not require the nurse's immediate attention. This is a normal manifestation after a bronchoscopy. The swallowing reflex is usually blocked for about six hours after the procedure. Initially, the client may have some discomfort and difficulty when the swallowing reflex is restored.*

4. **CORRECT. This is a priority assessment that needs immediate medical treatment. The difficulty in breathing may be caused by edema in the larynx or trachea and is a serious complication.**

57. **The nurse is caring for a client who had abdominal surgery two days ago. Which assessment data requires immediate action by the nurse?**

1. A urinary drainage bag with 100 mL in a two-hour period.
2. A wound dressing with thick, light green drainage.
3. A blood pressure reading of 98/66.
4. Shallow respirations, with a rate of 26.

1. *INCORRECT. This assessment data would not require any action by the nurse. The amount of urine in the drainage bag indicates adequate urinary output.*

2. **CORRECT. Thick, light green drainage is indicative of an infection and should be reported to the physician immediately. The stem of the question requires analysis of the data by the nurse. This option also addresses a client safety issue, which requires an immediate response by the nurse.**

3. *INCORRECT. Since baseline data is not provided in the question, the nurse cannot determine whether or not the blood pressure reading is normal for this client. Further assessment is needed.*

4. *INCORRECT. Shallow respirations are not unusual for the client who has undergone abdominal surgery. Although the nurse needs to address this issue by having the client deep breathe and cough, it is not the priority action.*

58. **A depressed client attends a client education class on the topic of depression and learn about the behaviors that could indicate a recurrence of depression. To evaluate the effectiveness of the teaching, the nurse asks the client to identify the indications of recurrence of depression. Which behavior or manifestation, if named by the client, would indicate to the nurse the need for further instruction?**

    1. Psychomotor retardation.
    2. Grandiosity.
    3. Self-devaluation.
    4. Insomnia.

    1. INCORRECT. Psychomotor retardation may be a sign of recurrence of depression. Look for the option that is NOT a sign of depression.

    2. CORRECT. Grandiosity is not associated with depression; it is associated with the manic phase of bipolar depression.

    3. INCORRECT. Self-devaluation is associated with depression. Look for the option that is NOT a sign of depression.

    4. INCORRECT. Insomnia or hypersomnia are two interrupted sleep patterns that are associated with depression. This false response question is asking for an option that is NOT a sign of depression.

59. **An 18-month-old child is admitted for a surgical repair of the cleft palate. The child returns from the operating room supine, with an IV and a mist tent on room air. Which is the priority nursing action?**

    1. Medicate for pain.
    2. Check the IV for signs of infiltration.
    3. Turn the child on the side.
    4. Review the postoperative orders.

    1. INCORRECT. The child may need medication for pain at some point, but this is not of immediate concern. TEST-TAKING TIP: This is a prioritizing question; choose the option the nurse should do first.

    2. INCORRECT. The IV site should be checked frequently to ensure patency and placement, but this is not of immediate concern. TEST-TAKING TIP: This is a prioritizing question; choose the option the nurse should do first.

    3. CORRECT. Airway is always an immediate priority. Turning the child on the side will protect the child from aspiration.

    4. INCORRECT. The postoperative orders should be reviewed when the child is admitted to the acute care floor. This would not take precedence, however, over establishing a patent airway in a child at risk for aspiration. TEST-TAKING TIP: This is a prioritizing question; choose the option the nurse should do first.

60. **A male nurse receives a doctor's order to catheterize one of his female clients. The client says, "I'm not going to allow a male nurse to catheterize me." The appropriate response by the nurse is:**

    1. "Your doctor is a male. Would you let him catheterize you?"
    2. "I've done this many times with no problems."
    3. "You can explain to your doctor why the catheter wasn't inserted."
    4. "You appear to be upset. Let me find a female nurse to help with the procedure."

    1. INCORRECT. This response is defensive, focuses on an inappropriate person (the doctor), focuses on an inappropriate issue (whether the client would allow the doctor to catheterize her), and devalues the client's feelings. This response places the client on the defensive and is not therapeutic.

    2. INCORRECT. This response is defensive, focuses on an inappropriate person (the nurse), focuses on an inappropriate issue (the nurse's competency), and does not address the client's feelings or concerns. This response is not therapeutic for the client.

    3. INCORRECT. This response is defensive, focuses on an inappropriate person (the doctor) and aggravates the problem. With this response, the nurse will fail to see that the required procedure is performed, which might endanger the client. This response is not professional.

    4. CORRECT. This response shows empathy, responds to the client's concern and offers a possible solution to the problem. This is the best of the four options for this question. The other options are defensive, not client-centered, and do not respect client rights.

61. **A confused elderly client is found wandering around the ward wearing a bathrobe and cotton socks. The client is bumping into walls while walking. At this time, the nurse should:**

    1. Bring the client's shoes and help the client put them on.
    2. Accompany the client back to the room and obtain a baseline assessment.
    3. Ask the client to return to the room and rest until feeling better.
    4. Tell the client to be careful of any wet spots on the floor.

    1. INCORRECT. In this option, the nurse fails to ensure the client's immediate safety. The client is at risk of falling because of ambulating in stocking feet and bumping into walls. This option also does not address the issue of what is causing the client to bump into walls.

    2. CORRECT. The nurse ensures safety by accompanying the client back to the client's room. Assessment is also essential because the client's bumping into walls indicates impairment of the client's balance and level of consciousness, which may be a manifestation of an emerging complication.

    3. INCORRECT. In this option, the nurse fails to ensure the client's immediate safety. Also, the nurse does not know if the client feels ill or will feel better later. The nurse needs more information.

4. *INCORRECT. The case scenario does not tell you anything about wet spots on the floor, and this option does not address the issue of the client's bumping into walls. The nurse must act to provide for the client's immediate safety, and the nurse needs more information to determine the cause of the client's behavior.*

62. **A conscious client is brought to the emergency room after an automobile accident. A physical examination and x-rays reveal a transection of the spinal cord at T-4. The nurse should give the highest priority to which information? The client:**

1. Has an allergy to iodine.
2. Last voided seven hours ago.
3. Smokes two packs of cigarettes a day.
4. Is menstruating.

1. *INCORRECT. Although this information may be important later, especially if any diagnostic tests using dye contrast media are ordered, it is not priority at this time. Look for an option that can be life-threatening to the client in this immediate situation.*
2. **CORRECT. This is the priority information. A distended bladder is the most common cause of autonomic dysreflexia, an acute emergency that occurs as a result of exaggerated autonomic responses. It is characterized by severe, pounding headache with paroxysmal hypertension, profuse sweating, and bradycardia. Because this is an emergency situation, the objective is to remove the triggering stimulus as soon as possible.**
3. *INCORRECT. This assessment is certainly important to validate the high risk for respiratory complications secondary to smoking; however, it's not the priority observation at this time. Look for an option that can be life-threatening to the client in this immediate situation.*
4. *INCORRECT. The fact that the client is menstruating does not constitute an immediate emergency situation.*

63. **A female client is taking ampicillin (Amcill) and birth control pills containing estrogen. What information should the nurse provide?**

1. Take both medications with breakfast to avoid gastric upset.
2. When used together, serum potassium levels may rise.
3. The effectiveness of the birth control pills may be reduced while the client is taking ampicillin.
4. Urticaria is much more common when antibiotics are given with other drugs.

1. *INCORRECT. This would not be advisable because the effect of ampicillin is decreased slightly when taken with foods.*
2. *INCORRECT. Potassium levels are only monitored with IV penicillins that contain high amounts of potassium, such as Potassium Pen G.*

3. **CORRECT. The issue in this question is drug interaction. Estrogen metabolism is increased, or there is a reduction of enterohepatic circulation of estrogens, when ampicillin is taken by a woman using birth control pills. Another form of birth control should be used while a client is on ampicillin.**
4. *INCORRECT. Urticaria occurs with sensitivities to all penicillins, regardless of whether another medication is being used. This option does not address the issue in the question, which is drug interaction.*

64. **A client is admitted to the hospital for surgery after finding a lump in his right testicle. He asks the nurse, "Do you think the doctor will find cancer?" What is the best nursing response?**

1. "Most lumps found in the testicles are benign."
2. "It must be difficult for you not to know what the doctor will find."
3. "I think that you should discuss this with your doctor."
4. "It might be, but the doctor won't know until the surgery is performed."

1. *INCORRECT. This may be a true statement, but it does not allow the client to express his fears concerning cancer. This response blocks communication between the client and the nurse.*
2. **CORRECT. This is the best response by the nurse because it promotes communication by allowing the client to express his feelings.**
3. *INCORRECT. Referring the client's concern to the doctor puts the client's concern on hold and is not a therapeutic nursing response. The client's feelings and concerns need to be addressed by the nurse.*
4. *INCORRECT. This response does not help the client to explore his feelings and is not a therapeutic nursing response.*

65. **A client's psychiatrist orders lithium (Lithane) four times daily. When administering medications on the sixth day, the nurse notes that the client's laboratory report indicates a serum lithium level of 1.0 mEq/liter. Based on this lab report, the most appropriate nursing action at this time is to:**

1. Withhold the next dose of lithium and notify the psychiatrist.
2. Ask that the laboratory test be repeated.
3. Assess the client for possible toxic effects.
4. Administer the next dose of lithium as ordered.

1. *INCORRECT. This is an inappropriate action because the lithium level is within the therapeutic range.*
2. *INCORRECT. This is not necessary becaus the lithium level is within the therapeutic range.*
3. *INCORRECT. Since the nurse should continuously assess the client's responses to medication. this is an appropriate nursing action. It is not, however, an action that the nurse would take "based on the lab report," because the report indicates that the lithium level is within the therapeutic range. The case scenario presents no information suggesting lithium toxicity. Do not "read into" the question-and be sure to read all the options before identifying the best one.*

*4. CORRECT. The lithium level is within the thera-
peutic range. The next dose should be administered as ordered.*

> TEST-TAKING TIP: If you could not select the correct op-
> tion using your nursing knowledge alone, you could use
> the strategy of eliminating similar distractors in this ques-
> tion. Note that Options 1, 2, and 3 would be appropriate
> only if the level were outside the therapeutic range. Op-
> tion 4 is the option that is different. This strategy is useful
> to know.

66. A client is seen in the clinic in the 28th week of gestation.
Her blood pressure is 160/100 and she has 2+ protein
in her urine. Her doctor recommends hospitalization.
Because each available room on the unit is a semiprivate room, the client must share a room. The nurse
knows the appropriate roommate for this client is a:

1. 20-year-old primigravida who enjoys loud rock-and-
roll music.
2. 32-year-old multigravida who enjoys reading romance novels.
3. 24-year-old C-section who watches soap operas and
game shows on TV.
4. 22-year-old primigravida who has many visitors during the afternoon and evening.

*1. INCORRECT. The client has manifestations of preec-
lampsia, including hypertension, proteinuria, and
ankle edema. Because of the hypertension and danger of seizures, the best environment for her is one
that will facilitate rest and relaxation. The roommate in this option will increase the noise in the
environment. The same is true of the roommates in
Options 3 and 4, and these similar distractors should
be eliminated.*

*2. CORRECT. The client has manifestations of
preeclampsia, including hypertension, proteinuria, and ankle edema. Because of the hypertension, there is a danger of seizures. The
best environment for her is one that will facilitate rest and relaxation. A roommate who likes
quiet activities such as reading will be best.*

> TEST-TAKING TIP: In each of the other three options, the
> roommate will increase the noise in the environment. These
> similar distractors should all be eliminated.

*3. INCORRECT. The client has manifestations of preec-
lampsia, including hypertension, proteinuria, and ankle
edema. Because of the hypertension and danger of
seizures, the best environment for her is one that will
facilitate rest and relaxation. The roommate in this
option will increase the noise in the environment. The
same is true of the roommates in Options 1 and 4, and
these similar distractors should be eliminated.*

*4. INCORRECT. The client has manifestations of preec-
lampsia, including hypertension, proteinuria, and
ankle edema. Because of the hypertension and danger of seizures, the best environment for her is one
that will facilitate rest and relaxation. The roommate in this option will increase the noise in the
environment. The same is true of the roommates in
Options 1 and 3, and these similar distractors should
be eliminated.*

67. A client asks the nurse how relaxation techniques
will help reduce gastric pain. The client asks, "Can't
I just take the cimetidine (Tagamet) that my physician has prescribed?" In responding to this question, the nurse is guided by the knowledge that:

1. Gastric ulcer is a stress-related illness, and the
client's stress levels and emotional issues are contributing to the exacerbation of the manifestations.
2. The client is in denial, because the client is refusing
to acknowledge the role stress plays in the progress
of this illness.
3. Gastric ulcer and other psychosomatic illnesses are
caused by stress and cannot be cured with only
medical or surgical treatments.
4. The client is displaying the "typical ulcer personality" of a competitive, aggressive person who is defending against unresolved dependency needs.

*1. CORRECT. The client's question indicates that
the client does not readily perceive the relationship between stress and the exacerbation
of the ulcer. The nurse, guided by this knowledge, can formulate a response to help the client better understand the illness.*

*2. INCORRECT. The client's question does not neces-
sarily indicate denial. Without additional assessment
data not presented in this case scenario, the nurse
cannot know whether the client is refusing to acknowledge the role of stress in the illness. Do not
"read into" the question.*

*3. INCORRECT. Stress alone does not cause a gastric
ulcer. There are physiological factors that are more
directly involved.*

*4. INCORRECT. Current research indicates that a "typi-
cal ulcer personality" does not exist.*

68. A six-week-old infant with AIDS is being prepared
for discharge. The infant's primary caregiver is
the grandmother. Which statement by the grandmother would alert the nurse to a need for further
instruction?

1. "I know that handwashing is an important preventative measure."
2. "I'll use disposable diapers, discarding them in
sepaprioritizing question—what is the most important nursing goal?

*1. INCORRECT. This statement does not represent a
hazard. It indicates the grandmother's understanding of transmission of the disease and the effectiveness of handwashing as an effective method of preventing infection to the client and to the family. This
is an appropriate response, however, the question
is asking you to identify an inappropriate response.*

*2. INCORRECT. This is an acceptable method of infec-
tion control. Any items that cannot be disposed of in
the toilet should be kept in a closed plastic bag until
trash disposal. This statement by the grandmother
does not represent a knowledge deficit. The question
is asking you to identify an inappropriate response.*

3. **CORRECT. This is an inadequate method of cleaning blood or potentially contaminated body substances. Bleach solution should be used and gloves worn whenever coming in contact with blood or other body substances. This answer is correct because the question asks you to identify the inappropriate response.**

4. *INCORRECT. This is an appropriate response by the grandmother because gloves should be worn by anyone when changing the diaper of a child who has tested HIV positive or has the AIDS virus. Blood and body fluids are a means of disease transmission. The question is asking you to identify an inappropriate response.*

69. **The most important nursing goal for a client who is admitted with an acute exacerbation of ulcerative colitis is to:**

    1. Provide emotional support.
    2. Prevent skin breakdown.
    3. Maintain fluid and electrolyte balance.
    4. Promote physical rest.

    1. *INCORRECT. Emotional support is necessary, but physiological needs must be the priority in the acute stage. This is a prioritizing question—what is the most important nursing goal?*

    2. *INCORRECT. Preventing skin breakdown is important, but this is not the "most important nursing goal" for this client. This is a prioritizing question—what is the most important nursing goal?*

    3. *CORRECT. This is the most important nursing goal in this case. Problems related to fluid and electrolyte balance can affect all systems. The primary goal would be to treat imbalances.*

    4. *INCORRECT. Rest promotes a decreased metabolic rate, but it is not sufficient to counteract problems resulting from fluid and electrolyte imbalances. This is a prioritizing question—what is the most important nursing goal?*

70. **The nurse observes an elderly client trying to climb over the side rails of the bed. The nurse is placing a vest restraint on the client when the daughter arrives and says to the nurse, "My parent does not need to be tied down in bed. I've been taking care of my parent for years, and my parent hasn't fallen out of bed yet." The initial response by the nurse is:**

    1. "I just saw your parent trying to climb over the side rails. Since I am concerned about your parent falling and getting hurt, I think this is best for safety."
    2. "Tell me how you managed to care for your parent at home."
    3. "Hospital policy requires restraint vests on clients who are at risk for falling. I just saw your parent trying to climb over the rails. You don't want your parent to get hurt, do you?"
    4. "The elderly may become confused in an unfamiliar place and do things they wouldn't do at home. It is difficult to see your parent restrained. While you are with your parent, the restraints can be off. Let me know when you are ready to leave."

1. *INCORRECT. The client's safety is the issue in this question. Since the daughter and nurse are with the parent, there is no immediate danger. It is important to note that the client in this test question is the daughter, and the nurse should address the daughter's statement. This response focuses on safety and restraints, and not on the client's (the daughter's) concerns about her parent being tied down.*

2. *INCORRECT. This option may be appropriate later in the conversation, but is not the initial response. This response does not focus on the issue in the question, which is the client's feelings about restraints being placed on her parent.*

3. *INCORRECT. This response implies that the daughter is not interested in her parent's safety and makes her defensive. It focuses on hospital policy and not the daughter's concerns. The daughter is the client in this question, and the nurse's response must be therapeutic for the daughter.*

4. **CORRECT. This option focuses on the daughter's concerns. It uses the therapeutic communication tool 1. CORRECT. The client's nutritional status should receive first priority, because nutrition is a basic physiological need. If the client's nutritional needs are not met, the situation may be life-threatening. TEST-TAKING TIP: Remember the nursing process—assess first!**

71. **The nurse is caring for a client who is recovering from surgery. The client has a urinary catheter in place that needs to be irrigated. The nurse knows the correct approach to prevent injury to the mucosa of the bladder is:**

    1. Gently compress the ball of the syringe to instill the irrigating solution.
    2. Quickly instill the irrigating solution, using some pressure to loosen any clots or mucous.
    3. After instilling the solution, apply gentle pressure to remove the irrigating solution from the bladder.
    4. Place a sterile cap on the end of the drainage tubing to protect it from contamination.

    1. **CORRECT. Gentle instillation creates a flow that helps to dilute and free sediment or debris within the lumen of the catheter.**

    2. *INCORRECT. Using force can injure tissue or cause the solution to leak from the connection. Any suction should be avoided because the mucosa of the bladder is easily injured. Removing the syringe from the catheter will break any suction created by vacuum. Note that Option 3 also involves the use of "pressure." Both of these options are wrong.*

    3. *INCORRECT. Using force can injure the mucosa of the bladder. Like Option 2, this distractor involves "pressure." This is a clue that both of these similar distractors are wrong.*

    4. *INCORRECT. A sterile cap can help prevent a potential infection but does not protect the mucosa of the bladder from injury during irrigation. This option does not address the issue in the question.*

72. A client is admitted to the hospital because of extreme weight loss. It is noted on the admission assessment that the client feels overweight at 88 pounds. What aspect of care should the nurse consider the first priority for this client's care?

1. Assessing the client's nutritional status.
2. Obtaining a psychiatric consult.
3. Planning a therapeutic diet for the client.
4. Talking to family members to find out more about the client's self-concept.

1. *CORRECT. The client's nutritional status should receive first priority, because nutrition is a basic physiological need. If the client's nutritional needs are not met, the situation may be life-threatening.* TEST-TAKING TIP: *Remember the nursing process—assess first!*
2. *INCORRECT. Obtaining a psychiatric consult may be an appropriate intervention, but with the limited information given in this case scenario, it would not take priority at this time.*
3. *INCORRECT. The client will need adequate nutrition and you are correct in identifying nutrition as a basic physiological need and a high priority. However, planning nursing interventions should come after one of the other options in this question.*
4. *INCORRECT. Obtaining further information from the family may be appropriate, but it is not the priority action in this situation.*

73. A client is hospitalized for a closed reduction of a fractured femur and application of a cast. A vital nursing action in the care of this client is to:

1. Perform neurovascular checks of the extremities.
2. Use the palms of the hands when moving an extremity with a wet cast.
3. Provide an instrument for the client to scratch the itching areas of skin under the cast.
4. Petal the edges of the cast to provide smooth edges.

1. *CORRECT. This is an important aspect of care for the client with a fracture. Circulation can become compromised and cause nerve and tissue damage. This action is more "vital" than the other three options.*
2. *INCORRECT. Using fingertips on a wet cast can cause indentations in the cast, resulting in pressure areas inside the cast. Therefore, using the palms instead of fingertips is an appropriate nursing action, but it is not the most important or "vital" action. Read all the options, and make another choice.*
3. *INCORRECT. This is not an appropriate nursing action. Scratching under the cast can cause injury to the skin and potential infection.*
4. *INCORRECT. Although petaling the edges of the cast should be done to prevent injury to the skin caused by uneven edges of the cast, this is not the most important or "vital" nursing action.*

74. After detoxification, a client begins the rehabilitation phase of treatment. The client tells the nurse, "I cannot imagine living my life without alcohol." The nurse's best response is based on the knowledge that the client:

1. Will be more successful if the client focuses on goals for short periods of time.
2. Is likely to drink again when under stress.
3. Will not be successful if the client is not strongly motivated.
4. May require treatment with Antabuse to maintain sobriety.

1. *CORRECT. Clients are less overwhelmed by the thought of sobriety when they set short-term goals that focus on "today" or "this week." Dealing with shorter periods of time is more manageable. The AA maxim, "One day at a time," is a reflection of this principle.*
2. *INCORRECT. While this might be true, it is not the basis for a therapeutic response for this client. What is the best response by the nurse?*
3. *INCORRECT. This is not the best option. Motivation, without the development of needed skills, will not help the client to maintain sobriety.*
4. *INCORRECT. Antabuse is used for individuals who lack the ability to abstain from alcohol without fear of adverse consequences. There is no data to indicate that this client requires Antabuse, since the client's rehabilitation program is just beginning. Do not "read into" the question.*

75. While performing a vaginal exam on an obstetrical client, the nurse notes a glistening white cord in the vagina. The first nursing action is to:

1. Return to the nurses' station to place an emergency call to the physician.
2. Start oxygen at six to 10 liters, and assess the client's vital signs.
3. Cover the cord with a sterile, moist saline dressing.
4. Apply manual pressure on the presenting part and have the mother get into a knee-chest position.

1. *INCORRECT. The physician needs to be called, but this is not the first priority—the health of the fetus is! What should the nurse do FIRST?*
2. *INCORRECT. This would not be helpful. All the oxygen in the world is not going to help this fetus if it cannot get it through the umbilical cord. The mother's vital signs are not a concern with a prolapsed cord; the fetal heart rate is of grave concern.*
3. *INCORRECT. This is not the best choice. Covering the cord with a moist sterile dressing will keep the cord moist and sterile, but it will not oxygenate the fetus. What should the nurse do FIRST?*
4. *CORRECT. This is the first nursing action because it is essential to get any pressure off the umbilical cord to allow oxygen to get to this fetus. Manual pressure on the presenting part and a knee-chest position are two ways to relieve umbilical cord compression.*

76. A client is in the hospital and has just found out that the parent died of a heart attack. The client is crying and has the face buried in a pillow. The most therapeutic nursing response at this time is to:

1. Return in fifteen minutes to see how the client is doing.
2. Sit with the client for a little while.
3. Tell the client that things will feel better in the morning.
4. Share with the client that the nurse knows just how the client feels because the nurse's parent recently died.

1. INCORRECT. This response does not promote therapeutic communication for the "here and now" of this question. The action indicates to the client that the nurse is not willing to offer self by staying during this stressful time. If the client wanted to communicate, there would not be anyone to listen.

2. CORRECT. The nurse lets the client know that the client's feelings are important by providing personal time. Being silent is a communication tool that is appropriate during times of grieving. This response also addresses the "here and now" in this question.

3. INCORRECT. This response devalues the client's feelings and puts them on hold. This response does not encourage therapeutic communication. It also offers false assurance, since the client may not feel better in the morning.

4. INCORRECT. This response focuses on an inappropriate person (the nurse) instead of on the client. When the nurse expresses complete understanding of how the client feels, it inhibits communication by implying there is no need for the client to express personal feelings. There is also an assumption by the nurse that grieving is the same for everyone.

77. A client with asthma is receiving an oxygen concentration of 35%. The nurse knows that achievement of the therapeutic goal of this treatment is best demonstrated by:

1. Absence of adventitious breath sounds.
2. PaO$_2$ 92.
3. Heart rate increase of 25 beats/min.
4. Bicarbonate level of 25 mEq/liter.

1. INCORRECT. This is not the best indicator of oxygen therapy treatment. The absence of adventitious breath sounds means that crackles and wheezing are not audible, but does not indicate if there is adequate gas exchange.

2. CORRECT. The goal of oxygen therapy is achievement of a PaO2 above 80 and no manifestations of oxygen toxicity. This is a good example of a test question that uses the evaluation phase of the nursing process.

3. INCORRECT. The opposite should occur if the oxygen is effective. The myocardial workload should be decreased, allowing for a slowing of the heart rate.

4. INCORRECT. The value given is a normal bicarbonate, but is not an indicator of the client's response to oxygen therapy. This value is used to detect acid-base deviations.

78. The primary nurse learns that an obsessive-compulsive client has a full set of dentures because the client's brushing rituals eroded all of the tooth enamel. The client also brushes the tongue several times a day, and has developed several ulcerations on it. The initial priority in the nursing care plan for this client is for the client to:

1. Eliminate the brushing and mouth care rituals.
2. Verbalize the underlying cause of this behavior.
3. Seek out the nurse when feeling anxious.
4. Reestablish healthy tissue in the mouth and tongue.

1. INCORRECT. While this option is the goal of the client's treatment, it is not the initial priority for the client's care. Look for the option that is the initial priority for the client.

2. INCORRECT. This may or may not be appropriate, as behavioral methods will most likely be used to treat the client's problems. Even if it is appropriate, this would not be the initial priority.

3. INCORRECT. This is an appropriate goal, but is not the initial priority for this client's care. Look for the option that is the initial priority for the client.

4. CORRECT. Restoring physiological integrity is the initial priority for this client. This will be done while working on the long-term goal of decreasing the mouth care rituals.

79. The nurse is informed during report that a postoperative client has not voided for eight hours. The initial nursing action is to:

1. Assist the client to the bathroom.
2. Place the client on a bed pan and pour warm water over the perineum.
3. Palpate and percuss the client's bladder.
4. Catheterize the client.

1. INCORRECT. Assisting the client to the bathroom may be helpful if the client needs to urinate. However, this information needs to be obtained before action is taken. TEST-TAKING TIP: Remember the nursing process—what is the initial nursing action?

2. INCORRECT. Placing the client on a bed pan is not always conducive to urinating. If the client is allowed out of bed, sitting on the toilet while pouring warm water over the perineum can facilitate the client to void. However, this is not the priority action. The client should have the need and an urge to void before this intervention is implemented.

3. CORRECT. Assessing the client's bladder provides information concerning the need to void. This is the priority action and the only option that provides for assessment of the client. TEST-TAKING TIP: Remember the nursing process—the nurse must assess first.

4. *INCORRECT. Catheterizing the client should only be done after it has been determined that the client has a full bladder and is unable to void. TEST-TAKING TIP: Remember the nursing process—the nurse must assess first.*

80. **A three-year-old is being admitted with nephrotic syndrome. The best roommate the nurse can select for this client is:**

    1. A 16-year-old recovering post-operatively from a ruptured appendix.
    2. An eight-year-old with leukemia.
    3. Another toddler with rheumatic fever.
    4. No roommate because isolation is required.

    1. *INCORRECT. The child with nephrotic syndrome is at risk for infection.*
    2. **CORRECT. This child is not infectious, which is what the nurse is looking for as a roommate for a child with nephrotic syndrome. The roommates may have nothing in common, but the potential for infection is a high priority nursing diagnosis for this admission.**
    3. *INCORRECT. The child with rheumatic fever may still be infectious from the original causative organism, and the child with nephrotic syndrome is at risk for infection.*
    4. *INCORRECT. It is not necessary to place this child on isolation.*

81. **A client is to receive antibiotics. The priority nursing action when preparing to administer this medication is to:**

    1. Determine if the client has any allergies.
    2. Determine the route of administration.
    3. Check the client's name band.
    4. Check the dosage against the physician's order.

    1. **CORRECT. An allergy to an antibiotic can cause serious side effects. This is the priority nursing action, since the safety of the client is the issue.**

    > **TEST-TAKING TIP:** This option assesses before implementing. Use the nursing process when answering test questions.

    2. *INCORRECT. This is an incorrect response because this is not a nursing action. The physician determines the route of administration, while the nurse implements the order. If there is a question about the route, the nurse needs to clarify the order. Which of the options represents the priority nursing action?*
    3. *INCORRECT. It is true that the client's name band should be checked before administering any medication. However, the priority nursing action in preparing to administer the medication is to note any allergies, especially when the medication is an antibiotic. Remember, safety first!*
    4. *INCORRECT. This is an appropriate action, but it is not the priority here. Determining that the dose is correct is a nursing standard for medication preparation. If the client is allergic to the medication, however, the nurse need not prepare it. Notifying the physician of this fact is the next step and the priority nursing action.*

82. **Before administering lithium, the nurse checks the client's latest lab report for the serum lithium level and notes a level of 1.2 mEq/L. What is the best action for the nurse to take next?**

    1. Administer the next prescribed dose of lithium.
    2. Suggest the blood test be repeated.
    3. Withhold the next dose of lithium and notify the psychiatrist of the lab results.
    4. Ask the client how he is feeling, to identify any untoward effects.

    1. *INCORRECT. Although this action is a possibility, it could be unsafe. The lithium level is still within the therapeutic range, but it is at the very top of the range. Read the other options to see if there is a better choice.*
    2. *INCORRECT. This action could be appropriate, but it is not the best action for the nurse to take next. Read the other options.*
    3. *INCORRECT. This is a not correct action. The lithium level is still within the normal range, so withholding the lithium is not an appropriate nursing action.*
    4. **CORRECT. A lithium level of 1.2 mEq/L is at the top of the therapeutic range. Before the nurse can safely give the next dose, the client must be assessed for any signs of lithium toxicity. If the client has none, the medication can be given as prescribed.**

83. **A client is admitted to the psychiatric unit with a diagnosis of acute depression. After being hospitalized for a few weeks, the client says to the nurse, "I'm a terrible person, and I should be dead." The nurse understands that the initial response would be:**

    1. "That is why you are here. We are trying to help you with your bad feelings."
    2. "Feeling that way must be awful. What makes you feel so terrible?"
    3. "Feeling like a terrible person is part of your illness. As you get better, those feelings will lessen."
    4. "You are not terrible. You are not a bad person."

    1. *INCORRECT. This response is not therapeutic because it appears to support the client's feelings of being a terrible person. The second part of the response also blocks therapeutic communication by focusing on inappropriate persons: the nurse and others who "are trying to help" the client.*
    2. **CORRECT. This response shows empathy, and then seeks clarification of the client's feelings. These two communication tools combine to make a therapeutic response that allows the client discuss any feelings.**
    3. *INCORRECT. This is not the initial response because it only gives information about the illness. At this time, the client's feelings must be addressed before information is given. When a client is distressed and upset, giving an explanation is inappropriate.*
    4. *INCORRECT. This response is not therapeutic for the client. The nurse's opinion is not important. This response blocks therapeutic communication by putting the nurse in the role of an authority figure, using false reassurance, and devaluing the client's feelings. The nurse's response should encourage the client to explore the feelings with the nurse.*

84. The nurse in a long-term care facility finds an elderly client on the floor. After having the client examined by the physician, the most important nursing action is to:

1. Call the family to stay with the client.
2. Provide for the safety and protection of the client.
3. Apply wrist and leg restraints to prevent the client from falling out of bed.
4. Obtain an order for medication to sedate the client.

1. INCORRECT. Having a member of the family stay with the client may be a possibility if it can be arranged. This provides for the client's safety and allows some mobility for the client while in bed. However, this is not the best option.

2. CORRECT. This global response option includes providing all appropriate interventions that address the safety needs of the client. Maslow's hierarchy of needs indicates that the client's safety receives highest priority when no basic physiologic need is identified.

3. INCORRECT. This is not the correct answer because wrist and leg restraints are not the first nursing action. Application of restraints may be appropriate to ensure the safety of the client. A vest restraint would be more appropriate, however, since it provides mobility for the client and is less likely to cause agitation of the client.

4. INCORRECT. Other measures should take priority over sedation. Sedating a client often makes the client more confused and more likely to behave inappropriately.

85. A client was admitted one week ago with a diagnosis of schizophrenia, paranoid type. Since admission, the client has had several verbal outbursts of anger but has not been violent. A staff member tells the nurse that the client is pacing up and down the hall very rapidly and muttering in an angry manner. The initial nursing action is to:

1. Prepare an intramuscular injection of haloperidol (Haldol) to give the client p.r.n.
2. Observe the behavior and approach the client in a non-threatening manner.
3. Gather several staff members and approach the client together.
4. Contact the client's psychiatrist and request an order to place the client in seclusion.

1. INCORRECT. This is not the initial nursing action. While a p.r.n. dose of an antipsychotic may be necessary if the client is unable to control behavior, the nurse needs more information at this time.

2. CORRECT. The nurse must first assess the client's condition before deciding on an appropriate intervention. The initial action is to approach calmly in a non-threatening manner, and ask the client to verbalize what is causing these upsetting feelings. Remember the nursing process—the nurse must always assess first.

3. INCORRECT. Although it is important to have sufficient staff available to handle a potentially unsafe situation, there is a better option that more specifically addresses the approach the nurse should take initially.

4. INCORRECT. This is not correct. The case scenario does not indicate that this intervention is needed.

86. Betamethasone (Celestone) is administered to a client at 30 weeks gestation to reduce the risk of respiratory distress syndrome (RDS) in the neonate. The infant is born after two injections are given. In planning nursing care for the infant, which finding should be anticipated as a result of the administration of betamethasone to the mother?

1. Rapid pulse rate.
2. Sternal retractions.
3. Hypoglycemia.
4. Hypothermia.

1. INCORRECT. Betamethasone administration given to the antepartum client does not have an effect on neonatal vital signs. If this neonate has a rapid apical pulse, it is related to another cause, most likely the prematurity.

2. INCORRECT. While it is quite likely that this premature neonate will have some RDS manifested by sternal retractions, it is most likely a result of immature lung development and not related to the administration of betamethasone.

3. CORRECT. Betamethasone causes hyperglycemia in the mother, which predisposes the neonate to hypoglycemia in the first hours after delivery. This question concerns the planning phase of the nursing process and requires a knowledge of pharmacokinetics.

4. INCORRECT. Betamethasone does not have any effect on the neonate's ability to maintain body temperature. If hypothermia is present, it is related to another cause, probably immature temperature regulation.

87. In preparing to begin an aminophylline (Phyllocontin) infusion, the best nursing approach would be:

1. Preparing a solution containing enough drug to last 24 hours.
2. Obtaining an infusion pump to regulate the flow of the drug.
3. Inserting a large IV catheter to assure adequate dilution.
4. Initiating measurement of intake and output to detect fluid retention.

1. INCORRECT. Since aminophylline can be very toxic if infused too quickly, the total daily dose should be divided into several IV containers. If the infusion rate increases, a limited amount of drug will be infused.

2. INCORRECT. Since aminophylline can be very toxic if infused too quickly, a pump should be used to regulate the flow of this drug.

> **TEST-TAKING TIP:** Note that the word "infusion" appears in the stem of the question and in this correct option. When you don't know the answer and other strategies do not apply (looking for a global response, and eliminating similar distractors), a repeated word or phrase can be a clue that this is the correct answer.

3. *INCORRECT. The size of the IV catheter is not relevant to dilution of the drug. The drug is diluted in the IV solution, not in the vein.*

4. *INCORRECT. Input and output should be monitored, but the nurse will be looking for dehydration rather than fluid retention, since aminophylline acts as a diuretic.*

88. **A client is being given an aminoglycoside for a bacterial infection. The nurse can aid in minimizing the risk of aminoglycoside toxicity by:**

1. Weighing the client daily.
2. Encouraging the client to drink at least 2,000 mL of fluids daily.
3. Monitoring blood pressure prior to drug administration.
4. Instructing the client to take the medicine with food.

1. *INCORRECT. Although daily weights are an assessment tool useful in monitoring fluid volume deficit or excess, this action doesn't directly address the major concern with aminoglycosides.*

2. ***CORRECT. Aminoglycosides accumulate in the kidneys, which is the site of excretion. Hydration serves to reduce the extent to which these drugs will be concentrated in the renal tubules, which can lead to renal toxicity. Remember that this intervention may be contraindicated in clients with a history of decreased renal function.***

3. *INCORRECT. Monitoring blood pressure is not necessary because hypertension is not a manifestation of aminoglycoside toxicity.*

4. *INCORRECT. Aminoglycosides are poorly absorbed from an intact intestinal tract, but are rapidly absorbed intramuscularly. The only oral uses of aminoglycosides are for surgical prophylaxis ("bowel sterilization") or treatment of intestinal infections.*

89. **A client is hospitalized for gastrointestinal bleeding and is being treated with temazepam (Restoril). After the physician examined the client, the nurse noted the physician wrote an order for the client to begin taking amitriptyline (Elavil). The initial action by the nurse is to:**

1. Revise the client's medication schedule so that the Elavil is administered during the day and the Restoril at bedtime.
2. Monitor the client's vital signs closely.
3. Question the physician about administering both Elavil and Restoril to the client.
4. Assess the client for manifestations of depression.

1. *INCORRECT. Elavil is a tricyclic antidepressant that is very sedating. It is often chosen for depressed clients who also have difficulty sleeping. Restoril, a benzodiazepine, potentiates the effect of Elavil. The issue in this question is drug interaction.*

2. *INCORRECT. This is not the best option. Although the client's vital signs should be monitored when placed on Elavil because it may cause orthostatic hypotension, this is not the initial nursing action in this case scenario. The issue in this question concerns drug interaction.*

3. ***CORRECT. Benzodiazepines, such as Restoril, potentiate the effects of other central nervous system depressants, such as the tricyclic Elavil. The nurse should contact the physician to question the safety of administering these two medications to the client.***

4. *INCORRECT. This is an appropriate nursing action, but it is not the best initial action. The issue in this question concerns a drug interaction. Review the choices again and select the better action.*

90. **The nurse is caring for a client with a myocardial infarction who is taking chlorothiazide (Diuril) and digoxin (Lanoxin). The most appropriate diet for the nurse to include in this client's nursing care is a diet:**

1. Low in sodium and saturated fats, high in potassium.
2. Low in unsaturated fats, sodium, and potassium.
3. High in potassium, Vitamin C, and protein.
4. Low in sodium and saturated and unsaturated fats.

1. ***CORRECT. Sodium would be restricted to decrease the circulating blood volume and reduce the cardiac workload. Saturated fats would be decreased to prevent further atherosclerotic heart disease. Potassium should be increased in the diet because Diuril causes the excretion of potassium in the urine. It is vital to keep potassium within normal limits because a low potassium level may lead to arrhythmias in a client who is taking digoxin.***

2. *INCORRECT. Both saturated and unsaturated fats are restricted in a weight reduction diet. However, the case scenario does not provide information that indicates this client needs to be placed on a weight reduction diet. Also, due to the drugs, loss of potassium can present a problem. Adequate potassium is needed to prevent cardiac arrhythmias.*

3. *INCORRECT. A diet high in potassium is needed because of the loss of potassium due to digoxin and Diuril. There is no reason for increasing Vitamin C or protein.*

4. *INCORRECT. Both saturated and unsaturated fats are restricted in a weight reduction diet, however, the case scenario does not provide information that indicates this client needs to be placed on a weight reduction diet. Also, due to the drugs, loss of potassium can present a problem. Adequate potassium is needed to prevent cardiac arrhythmias.*

91. **The nurse is caring for a client with diabetes who is currently taking cephalexin (Keflex). The nurse should advise the client that:**

1. Clinitest or copper sulfate urine glucose tests give false positive results.
2. Blood sugar may drop without warning.
3. A source of sugar should always be carried with the client.
4. A MedicAlert bracelet should always be worn.

1. *CORRECT. Cephalexin causes false positive results in urine glucose tests using cupric sulfate. Diabetic clients receiving cephalexin should use glucometers, or glucose enzymatic tests such as Clinistix.*
2. *INCORRECT. A drop in blood sugar is not a reaction caused by antibiotics.*
3. *INCORRECT. This precaution is appropriate for all diabetics, regardless of whether they are on any medications. Look for an answer that relates to the effect of cephalexin on diabetics, which is the issue in the question.*
4. *INCORRECT. All diabetics should wear a MedicAlert bracelet. This, however, does not address this client's need for advice regarding the effects of cephalexin.*

92. **An elderly client is admitted to the psychiatric unit for a diagnostic work-up because of increased forgetfulness and disorientation at home. The client has been taking lorazepam (Ativan) 0.5 mg p.r.n. to control restlessness. In planning nursing care for this client, it would be unnecessary to include close observation for:**

1. Orthostatic hypotension.
2. Increased anxiety.
3. Hyperexcitation.
4. Hallucinations.

1. *CORRECT. Orthostatic hypotension is a side effect of antipsychotics and tricyclic antidepressants. It is NOT a side effect of the benzodiazepines, like Ativan. This is the correct option because the stem is asking for an INCORRECT response.*
2. *INCORRECT. Increased anxiety is one of the manifestations of paradoxical excitement that can occur in elderly clients, so the nurse should closely observe for signs of increased anxiety. The stem in this question is asking for an INCORRECT response.*
3. *INCORRECT. Hyperexcitation is one of the manifestations of paradoxical excitement that can occur in elderly clients. This cannot be the correct option because the stem is asking for the manifestation that does NOT occur with Ativan.*
4. *INCORRECT. Hallucinations are one of the manifestations of paradoxical excitement that can occur in elderly clients. It is not the correct option. Select the manifestation that does NOT occur with Ativan.*

93. **A client with chronic emphysema is taking theophylline (Theo-Dur) at home. During the home care nurse's visit, which statement by the client would warrant immediate action?**

1. "I just lie awake at night, worrying about the medical bills."
2. "I must have the flu. I was vomiting all night."
3. "I don't have my usual appetite. Nothing tastes good to me."
4. "I feel better if I have a big glass of milk with my pill."

1. *INCORRECT. This statement does not warrant immediate action by the nurse. Insomnia is a common side effect of theophylline. While it is annoying and interferes with the client's rest, it is not life-threatening and does not call for immediate action.*
2. *CORRECT. While the client may indeed have the flu, one of the early signs of theophylline toxicity is vomiting. Since there is no antidote for theophylline, and since toxicity can be fatal, the nurse should immediately explore other possible signs of toxicity and request a serum theophylline level.*
3. *INCORRECT. This statement does not warrant immediate action by the nurse. A client receiving theophylline may have anorexia as a side effect of the drug. The client's nutritional status should be monitored. However, loss of appetite does not pose a life-threatening situation.*
4. *INCORRECT. This statement indicates that the client understands how to minimize the gastric irritation caused by theophylline. There is no reason why milk cannot be taken with theophylline.*

94. **A client is admitted to the psychiatric unit with a diagnosis of acute psychotic reaction. Because of extreme agitation, the client is started on chlorpromazine (Thorazine) 100 mg t.i.d. After three days, the client is much calmer and the nurse begins to teach the client about this medication. Which statement by the nurse is most appropriate?**

1. "This medication is a sedative to calm you down."
2. "This medication acts on the chemical regulators in your brain to help control your manifestations."
3. "This medication will cure your disorder."
4. "We do not know how this medication works, but we do know it will help you control your behavior."

1. *INCORRECT. This is not an accurate statement. Antipsychotic medications like Thorazine may calm an agitated client, but they are not sedatives. They also control other manifestations of psychosis, such as delusions and other thought disturbances.*
2. *CORRECT. Antipsychotic medications are thought to act directly on the dopamine receptors in the brain to prevent the re-uptake of dopamine and thereby control psychotic manifestations.*
3. *INCORRECT. This is not an accurate statement. Antipsychotics control manifestations but do not cure the psychotic disorder.*

4. *INCORRECT. This is only partially correct. The exact mechanisms of action are unknown, but research has provided some information about how these drugs work. Antipsychotics block dopamine receptors in the brain, thereby controlling the target manifestations of psychosis. Read the options again to identify a better nursing response.*

95. **A client is to have surgery the next day to create an ileal conduit and is receiving neomycin sulfate (Mycifradin Sulfate). The nurse's best explanation to the client for receiving neomycin preoperatively is that it:**

1. Suppresses intestinal bacteria preoperatively, to decrease the risk of postoperative infection.
2. Decreases the number of pathogenic bacteria and decreases the number of loose stools.
3. Sterilizes the bowel and prevents the risk of serious postoperative complications.
4. Prevents auditory impairment and nephrotoxicity during the postoperative period.

1. ***CORRECT. Because bowel contents may spill during the bowel resection, suppression of intestinal bacteria is done preoperatively to reduce the risk of postoperative infection.***
2. *INCORRECT. While neomycin is sometimes used to treat diarrhea caused by Escherichia coli, there is no data to support this rationale for this client. Be careful not to "read into" the question. The issue is the preoperative use of neomycin in a client scheduled for an ileal conduit. Look for the option that correctly addresses that issue.*
3. *INCORRECT. This explanation is incorrect. Living tissue cannot be sterilized; some organisms will remain.*
4. *INCORRECT. This answer does not make sense. Ototoxicity and nephrotoxicity are serious side effects of long-term neomycin treatment.*

96. **A client is admitted with pneumocystis carinii pneumonitis. The physician prescribes sulfamethoxazole trimethoprim (Bactrim), and a Foley catheter is inserted to monitor urinary output. Which nursing intervention would be most effective in reducing the risk of crystalluria secondary to sulfonamide therapy?**

1. Encouraging fluid intake to 3,000 mL/24 hours.
2. Irrigating the Foley catheter with normal saline every eight hours.
3. Monitoring specific gravity of urine every eight hours.
4. Providing foods and fluids likely to maintain an acidic pH of the urine.

1. ***CORRECT. Maintenance of hydration ("natural irrigation") is the most effective intervention in preventing urinary stasis, which can lead to crystalluria. The client's output should be at least 1,500 mL/day.***

2. *INCORRECT. Irrigating a Foley catheter should never be a routine procedure because of the risk of infection created by interrupting a sterile system. There is a better and safer option.*
3. *INCORRECT. Monitoring the specific gravity of urine will give information regarding urine osmolality and the kidneys' ability to concentrate urine. It will not reduce the risk of crystalluria because it's only an assessment tool. Choose a more effective intervention.*
4. *INCORRECT. The urine pH should be alkaline. Liquids and foods that produce acid urine should be avoided.*

97. **A client is to receive IM methylergonovine (Methergine). In caring for the client, the nurse knows the administration of IM Methergine is contraindicated in a client:**

1. Who is experiencing boggy fundus one hour after a vaginal delivery.
2. With a large amount of vaginal bleeding following an abortion at 16 weeks.
3. With a history of previous postpartum hemorrhage in the recovery room.
4. Who has not delivered the placenta 20 minutes following the birth of the baby.

1. *INCORRECT. This situation is an indication for the use of IM Methergine. A boggy fundus following delivery is indicative of uterine atony, which is treated by using an oxytocic drug such as Methergine. This question has a false response stem; so look for a contraindication.*
2. *INCORRECT. This situation is an indication for the use of IM Methergine. A large amount of bleeding following an abortion usually indicates poor contractility of the uterus and is treated with an oxytocic drug. Remember, this question has a false response stem; so look for a contraindication.*
3. *INCORRECT. This situation is an indication for the use of IM Methergine. Clients with a history of previous postpartum hemorrhage are usually given an oxytocic drug prophylactically following subsequent deliveries. This question has a false response stem. Look for a contraindication.*
4. ***CORRECT. Methergine is contraindicated prior to the delivery of the placenta.***

98. **A client is receiving propranolol (Inderal) for anxiety. In reviewing the client's discharge plans, the nurse needs to emphasize that Inderal:**

1. Should be discontinued by gradually tapering it off over time.
2. Should not be taken during pregnancy.
3. Is contraindicated for clients with asthma.
4. Is a safe medication with no known adverse effects.

1. ***CORRECT. Rapid withdrawal from Inderal in cardiac clients has been associated with cardiac arrhythmias and sudden death. As a general rule, it is discontinued by gradually tapering it off over time, to avoid any adverse responses.***

2. *INCORRECT. This is a possibility, but it is not the best option. Most medications should be avoided during pregnancy, but there is no indication that the client in this question is contemplating child-bearing or is even female. "Reading in" as simple a fact as gender can lead you astray. There are many facts that, added to this question, could affect the nurse's priority in discharge teaching. Which option deals with a priority that can be true for every client on Inderal?*

3. *INCORRECT. This is a true statement, but it is not the best response to this question about discharge teaching. The client's physical health was evaluated prior to starting Inderal to rule out any contraindications. There is a more important point for the nurse to emphasize prior to the client's discharge.*

4. *INCORRECT. This is not an appropriate statement. While Inderal is a relatively safe medication, it does have adverse effects.*

99. **A client has been taking trifluoperazine (Stelazine) for five years to control paranoid thoughts. When the client's sibling comes to visit, the sibling tells the nurse, "I believe that all psychiatric medications are a form of 'chemical mind control'." The nurse's best response to the sibling will incorporate the information that antipsychotic medications:**

1. Act directly on specific neurotransmitters in the brain to control the client's psychotic manifestations.

2. Act to sedate the client, therefore preventing the client from engaging in behavior that may cause difficulty.

3. Are a cure for psychotic disorders, like schizophrenic reactions, and are therefore an important part of the client's treatment plan.

4. Have been in use for close to 30 years and are safe and effective drugs for clients who have problems like this client's.

1. **CORRECT. *This is the best response to the sibling. The specific mechanisms of action are still unknown, but research indicates that antipsychotics act directly on the dopamine receptors in the brain and thereby control many target manifestations of psychosis.***

2. *INCORRECT. This is partially correct. Antipsychotic drugs do sedate the client to some degree, but that is not their primary mode of action. Look again at the other options to select one that provides a better rationale.*

3. *INCORRECT. This is an untrue statement because there is no known cure for schizophrenic disorders at this time. Many clients with these diagnoses have a chronic illness. Treatment is focused on helping them attain their highest level of functioning using medication and psychosocial therapies.*

4. *INCORRECT. Although this is true, it is not the best rationale for the nurse to use in responding to the client's concern. Look over the options to select a better rationale.*

100. **Which measure would the nurse select as providing the most accurate determination of renal impairment secondary to administration of amphotericin B (Fungizone)?**

1. Intake and output.
2. Daily weights.
3. Serum creatinine levels.
4. Serial potassium levels.

1. *INCORRECT. This would not be the best means to determine renal function. Monitoring input and output can give clues to renal function but cannot accurately define the problem.*

2. *INCORRECT. Daily weights are not the best indicator of renal function, although they do serve as a monitoring tool for fluid volume status. .*

3. **CORRECT. *Measurement of serum creatinine is used to detect impaired renal function. Serum creatinine should be monitored every other day as the dosage of amphotericin B is increased to optimal level, and then weekly until the drug is discontinued. If serum creatinine increases to 3 mg/mL, the dosage of should be decreased or discontinued until renal function improves.***

4. *INCORRECT. There is another option that would give an earlier and more accurate clue to decreased renal function.*

Chapter 12

REVIEW OF TEST-TAKING STRATEGIES FOR THE NCLEX

Section I: Preparing for the NCLEX

A. What You Should Know About the NCLEX-RN Exam
   1. General information
      a. The first integrated exam was given in July 1982
      b. The purpose of the exam is to determine that a candidate is prepared to practice nursing safely
      c. The exam is designed to test essential knowledge of nursing and a candidate's ability to apply that knowledge to clinical situations
      d. The purpose of the new test plan is to bring the exam in line with current nursing behaviors (the nursing process and decision making)
      e. Exam is "pass/fail," and no other score is given
   2. Computerized Adaptive Testing
      a. Computer program continuously scores answers and selects questions suitable for each candidate's competency level for a more precise measurement of competency
      b. A higher weight is assigned to difficult questions so a passing score can be obtained by answering a lot of easier questions-or a smaller number of more difficult questions
      c. Special screen design is used
      d. Use the mouse to move the cursor on the screen to the desired location. Single-click your mouse to select an option as your answer.
      e. A drop-down calculator also is featured. Double-click your mouse

on the calculator icon, and the drop-down calculator will appear.

    f. After you have confirmed your selection, click on "next" to input your answer and proceed to the next screen.

    g. After you proceed to the next screen, you CANNOT go back to a previous question to change your answer.

3. Exam schedule

    a. Given year-round

    b. Retake policy: The exam can only be repeated every 90 days

4. Number of questions and time allowed

    a. No minimum amount of time; however, a candidate must answer a minimum of 75 test questions

    b. Maximum time is five hours, with a maximum of 265 test questions

    c. About one out of three candidates completes the exam in less than two hours; one in three will use the complete five hours

    d. The computer will automatically stop as soon as one of the following occurs:

        1) Candidate's measure of competency is determined to be above or below the passing standard

        2) Candidate has answered all 265 test questions

        3) Maximum amount of time (five hours) has expired

5. A candidate will pass by either:

    a. Answering 75 to 265 questions above the passing standard (the required weighted score) for all questions answered, within the time allowed; or

    b. Answering at least 75 questions within the time allowed and achieving the passing standard for the last 60 questions answered

SCREEN DESIGN

On the psychiatric unit, a nurse observes a client standing near a window and touching the glass. The client also mutters from time to time. Which comment by the nurse indicates the best understanding of the client's behavior?

☐ 1. "Why are you standing by the window and touching the glass?"

Case Scenario and Stem

☐ 2. "There you are. I came to see if you wanted to see the video we are showing on the unit?"

☐ 3. "What are you looking at through the window?"

Choices 1, 2, 3, and 4

☐ 4. "Are you hearing voices or seeing things?"

6. Types of questions
   a. The majority of questions are standard multiple choice
      1) Each question has four options
      2) The best option is the only correct answer
   b. Exam includes 15 unmarked experimental or "try-out" questions
   c. A small percentage of questions are alternate format questions including:
      1) Fill-in-the blank items
         a) Calculation items
         b) Ordered Response
      2) Hot Spot (point & click items)
      3) Multiple Response
      4) Charts, Tables, & Graphic Images
7. Exam procedure:
   a. Look for the BEST answer to each question
   b. It is not possible to skip questions or return to previous questions
   c. Mandatory 10-minute break after first two hours and after another one-and-one-half hours
   d. Scratch paper provided for calculations must be returned at end of exam
8. Structure of the test plan *
   a. Safe, Effective Care Environment
      1) Management of Care   13-19%
      2) Safety and Infection Control   8-14%
   b. Health Promotion and Maintenance   6-12%
   c. Psychosocial Integrity   6-12%
   d. Physiological Integrity
      1) Basic Care and Comfort   6-12%
      2) Pharmacological and
         Parenteral Therapies   13-19%
      3) Reduction of Risk Potential   13-19%
      4) Physiological Adaptation   11-17%
      Information courtesy of the National Council of State Boards Nursing, Inc., Test Plan 2004.

B. Schedule Your Study Time
   1. The minimum time for preparation is two hours a day for six to eight weeks
      a. Spend 1/3 of your time reviewing content
      b. Spend 2/3 of your time answering test questions
   2. For content review, use an NCLEX-RN exam review book such as this one, which outlines content
   3. Begin with areas that are most difficult for you, or the areas that are least familiar

4. For more detailed information on your difficult or less familiar areas, use a good nursing reference manual

5. Review medical-surgical, pediatric, women's health, and psychiatric nursing, as well as nursing management and alternate test item formats

6. Use a body systems approach for medical-surgical and pediatric nursing areas

7. When studying body systems and the associated diseases, remember to:

   a. Define the disease in terms of the pathophysiological process that is occurring

   b. Identify the client's early and late manifestations

   c. Identify the most important or life-threatening complications

   d. Define the medical treatment

   e. Identify and prioritize the nursing interventions associated with early and late manifestations

   f. Identify what the nurse teaches the client/family to prevent or adapt to disease

8. To schedule your study time:

   a. List the areas you need to review

   b. Count the number of days you have available to study

   c. Estimate the amount of time needed for each area

   d. On your calendar, write the area to review, the number of questions to answer, and the amount of time needed for each study day

C. Answer Many Questions

1. Answering questions will develop your test-taking skills

2. Use questions similar to those on the NCLEX exam

3. Answer a minimum of 3,000 test questions

4. Include answering test questions in your study plan. For example, answer 100 questions each day for a month.

5. If you are at high risk, answer 5,000 test questions

6. Use at least three different question-and-answer books, including MEDS Publishing's *Complete Q&A for the NCLEX-RN Exam*

7. An online question and answer program which mimics the NCLEX exam, such as MEDS' StarNurse Exam-A-Day Gold, will give you a more realistic experience with answering alternate test item format questions

D. Assess Your Progress

1. Each time you answer questions, check the number of questions you answered correctly

   a. If you answer less than 65% correctly, this is a warning signal! Spend lots of time reviewing content and answering more questions in this area of nursing.

   b. If you answer 65 to 75% correctly, your performance is average. Success in this area is uncertain. Continue working with this content until your score is above 75%. Work on building your confidence by answering more questions in this area.

    c. If you answer 75 to 85% correctly, your performance is very good. Only return to this area after you have at least 75% in all other areas. Feel confident.

    d. If you answer 85 to 95% correctly, your performance is superior. Don't waste time on this. Feel very confident.

2. For each wrong answer, identify why you answered wrong

    a. You may have answered a question wrong because you did not know the facts or got confused about the information

       1) Identify this as a content weakness

       2) Review the content again

    b. You may have answered a question wrong because you misread the question, did not understand what it was asking, or did not know how to select the best answer

       1) Identify this as a test-taking deficiency

       2) For further assistance with test-taking deficiencies, we recommend MEDS' *Think Like A Nurse Online Series*

3. Check the number of questions that you identified as difficult and went back to answer later. See how many of them you answered correctly.

Section II: Answering Questions

A. Identify the Critical Elements in the Question

  1. Identify the issue in the question

    a. The issue is the problem about which the question is asking

    b. The issue may be a:

       1) Drug: for example, digoxin (*Lanoxin*), furosemide (*Lasix*)

       2) Nursing problem: for example, alteration in comfort, potential for infection

       3) Behavior: for example, restlessness, agitation

       4) Disorder: for example, diabetes mellitus, ulcerative colitis

       5) Procedure: for example, glucose tolerance test, cardiac catheterization

  2. Identify the client in the question

    a. The client in the question is usually the person with the health problem

    b. The client in a test question may also be a relative or significant other or another member of the health care team with whom the nurse is interacting

    c. The correct answer to the question must relate to the client in the question

3. Look for the key words

    a. Key words focus attention on what is important

    b. Key words may appear in bold print

    c. Examples:

        1) During the early period, which of the following nursing procedures would be **best**?

        2) The nurse would expect to find which of the following characteristics in an **adult** diabetic?

        3) Which of the following nursing actions is **vital**?

        4) Which of the following nursing actions would be best **initially**?

4. Identify what the stem is asking and determine whether the question has a true response stem or false response stem

    a. Be clear about what the stem is asking before you look at the options

    b. If the question is not clear to you, rephrase it using your own words

    c. Determine whether the question has a true response stem or a false response stem

        1) True response stem

            a) Definition: A true response stem requires an answer that is a true statement

            b) Examples:

                (1) Which of these interpretations is most justifiable?

                (2) The nurse would demonstrate best judgment by taking which of the following actions?

                (3) The chief purpose of the drug is to:

                (4) The nurse should give immediate consideration to which of the following findings?

        2) False response stem

            a) Definition: A false response stem requires an answer that is a false statement

            b) Examples:

                (1) Which of the following nursing actions would be inappropriate?

                (2) Which of the following statements by the client would indicate a need for further instruction?

                (3) Which of the following describes incorrect placement of the hands during CPR?

                (4) Which of the following actions would place the client at risk?

B. Use a Selection Procedure to Eliminate Incorrect Options
1. Most NCLEX questions have four options. The correct answer is the BEST answer. The other three options are "distractors."
2. Distractors are options made to look like correct answers. They are intended to distract you from answering correctly.
3. As you read each of the four options, make a decision about it.
   a. This option is true (+)
   b. This option is false (–)
   c. I am not sure about this option (?)
4. If the stem is a true response stem:
   a. An option that is true (+) might be the correct answer
   b. An option that is false (–) is a distractor. Eliminate this option
   c. An option that you are not sure about (?) is possibly the correct answer
5. If the stem is a false response stem:
   a. An option that is true (+) is a distractor. Eliminate this option.
   b. An option that is false (–) may be the correct answer
   c. An option that you are not sure about (?) is possibly the correct answer
6. Do not return to options you have eliminated
7. If you are left with one option, that is your answer
8. If you are left with one (+) option and one (?) option, select the (+) option as your answer
9. If you are left with two (+) options, use strategies to select the best answer

C. Use Test-Taking Strategies When You Are Unable to Select the Best Option
1. The Global Response Strategy
   a. A global response is a general statement that may include ideas of other options within it
   b. Look for a global response when more than one option appears to be correct
   c. The global response option will probably be the correct answer
2. The Similar Distractors Strategy
   a. Similar distractors say basically the same thing using different words
   b. Since there is only one correct answer in a question, similar distractors must be wrong
   c. Eliminate similar distractors. Select for your answer an option that is different.

3. The Similar Word or Phrase Strategy
   a. When more than one option appears to be correct, look for a similar word or phrase in the stem of the question and in one of the four options
   b. The option that contains the similar word or phrase may be the correct answer
   c. Use this strategy after you have tried to identify a global response option and eliminated similar distractors

D. Answering Communication Questions
   1. The NCLEX exam includes many communication questions because the ability to communicate therapeutically is essential for safe practice
   2. Identify the critical elements as in all questions. Pay particular attention to identification of the client in the question. Remember that the answer must relate to the client.
   3. Learn to identify communication tools that enhance communication.
      a. Being silent: Nonverbal communication
      b. Offering self: "Let me sit with you."
      c. Showing empathy: "You are upset."
      d. Focusing: "You say that . . ."
      e. Restatement: "You feel anxious?"
      f. Validation/clarification: "What you are saying is . . .?"
      g. Giving information: "Your room is 423."
      h. Dealing with the here and now: "At this time, the problem is . . ."
   4. Learn to identify non-therapeutic communication blocks.
      a. Giving advice: "If I were you, I would . . ."
      b. Showing approval/disapproval: "You did the right thing."
      c. Using clichés and false reassurances: "Don't worry. It will be all right."
      d. Requesting an explanation: "Why did you do that?"
      e. Devaluing client feelings: "Don't be concerned. It's not a problem."
      f. Being defensive: "Every nurse on this unit is exceptional."
      g. Focusing on inappropriate issues or persons: "Have I said something wrong?"
      h. Placing the client's issues "on hold": "Talk to your doctor about that."
   5. When answering communication questions, select an option that illustrates a therapeutic communication tool. Eliminate options that illustrate non-therapeutic communication blocks.

E. Answering Questions that Focus on Setting Priorities
   1. Priority-setting questions ask the test taker to identify either what comes first, is most important, or gets the highest priority

2. Examples:
   a. What is the nurse's initial response?
   b. The nurse should give immediate consideration to which of the following?
   c. Which nursing action receives the highest priority?
   d. What should the nurse do first?
3. Use guidelines to help you to answer priority setting questions
   a. Maslow's Hierarchy of Needs indicates that physiological needs come first
   b. Maslow's Hierarchy of Needs indicates that when no physiological need is identified, safety needs come first
   c. Nursing Process indicates that assessment comes first
   d. Communication Theory indicates focusing on feelings first
   e. Teaching/Learning Theory indicates focusing on motivation first

Section III: Preparing for Exam Time

A. Plan for Everything
   1. Assemble everything you will need for the exam the night before:
      a. Identification: two IDs with signatures, including one with recent photograph
      b. Watch
      c. Several sharpened pencils (with erasers) for calculations
   2. Plan to arrive at the test site early:
      a. Know the route to the exam site
      b. Know how long it will take to get there
      c. Know where you will park and if you will need coins for a parking meter
   3. Pay close attention to your own physiological needs:
      a. Dress in layers
      b. Get a good night's sleep the night before the exam
      c. Eat a good breakfast
      d. Avoid stimulants and depressants
      e. Use the bathroom just before the exam
   4. During the exam:
      a. Listen to the instructions
      b. Pace yourself; don't spend too long on any one question
      c. Don't let yourself become distracted. Focus your attention on answering the questions.

    d. Go with your first choice. Use test-taking strategies only when you cannot decide between close options.

    e. Keep your thoughts positive!

B. Manage Your Anxiety Level

  1. Moderate levels of anxiety increase your effectiveness

  2. Don't cram the night before the exam

  3. Do something enjoyable and relaxing the night before the exam

  4. Learn and practice measures to manage your anxiety level during the exam as needed

    a. Take a few deep breaths

    b. Tense and relax muscles

    c. Tell yourself positive affirmations

    d. Visualize a peaceful scene

    e. Visualize your success

C. Test-Taking Tips

  1. Prepare comprehensively and be sure to be well rested for the exam

  2. Read each question carefully, identifying the critical elements. Each question must be answered in sequence, and you may not skip or go back to change your answers to any questions.

  3. Don't panic if the computer stops after a short time! It does not mean that you failed. The computer stops when the exam is able to determine with at least 95% certainty that you have demonstrated the ability, or inability, to practice safely at the minimal level of nursing competency.

  4. It is helpful to know that most students pass by answering a maximum of all 265 questions.

  5. If you are having difficulty choosing between the best two options, use the three test-taking strategies you learned in this review:

    a. Look for the global response option

    b. Eliminate similar distractors

    c. Look for similar words in the question and one of the options

  6. You should anticipate that the test questions will increase in difficulty

  7. Use your scratch paper wisely. Since you cannot review earlier questions to help recall previous facts, use the scratch paper provided for calculations to remember facts from previous questions. Sometimes, information from one question is helpful in answering another question.

  8. Don't panic if someone finishes before you! The test adapts to each candidate's level of ability, and it means that you may take longer to prove that you are capable of practicing competently at the beginning level of nursing.

  9. Keep a positive attitude! Remember that you have learned a great amount of nursing knowledge, and the exam is only designed to determine whether you are able to practice safely at the entry level.

Chapter 13

NCLEX ALTERNATE TEST ITEM FORMATS

Section I: Overview

A. NCLEX Item Types
1. Standard Multiple Choice Question
   a. Traditionally, the format of NCLEX questions
   b. Still the most commonly seen type of question on the NCLEX
   c. Has four options, only one of which is correct ("one best option")
   d. Mastering this format is critical to your success on the NCLEX.
2. As of April 2003, the NCLEX started including items other than standard multiple choice questions. These items are known as Alternate Test Item Formats.
   a. Fill-in-the-Blank
      1) Calculation
      2) Sequence
   b. Multiple Response
   c. Hot Spot
   d. Charts, Tables, Graphic Images
3. The average standard question takes 60 to 70 seconds to answer.
4. The average candidate will be administered only one or two of these alternate items.

POINTS TO REMEMBER:
   You should allot a slightly longer time for alternate test items.

Section II: Fill-in-the-Blank

A. Overview
1. Definition: Fill-in-the-blank items are a type of alternate item that will be primarily numerical. This type of question typically involves either solving a math problem or putting a list of options into the correct sequence.
2. Method of Answer: To answer these questions, you will need to type a number into the answer box on the screen.

B. Types
1. Calculation item
    a. This type of fill-in-the-blank question typically involves solving a math problem.
    b. Method of Answer: To answer these questions, you will need to type a number into the answer box on the screen.
    c. Read the question carefully. If you see the question is asking for the answer in a specific unit amount, it is not necessary to put units in your answer.

POINTS TO REMEMBER:
1. Write equation down on your scrap paper.
2. Be certain you are solving for the correct unit value!
3. Show all of your work.
4. Bring up drop-down calculator.
5. Double-check your work

GRAPHIC 13-1.
FILL-IN-THE-BLANK CALCULATION ITEM

There are 13 clients being seen in the emergency room and 5 clients in the waiting room. What is the total number of clients?

Type your answer in the box below.

| 18 |

2. Sequence item
   a. This type of fill-in-the-blank question requires you to put a list of options into the correct order.
   b. Method of Answer: To answer these questions, you will need to type a series of numbers into the answer box on the screen.
   c. Read the question carefully. Sequence items on the NCLEX may require you to put the options in the order that you would perform them, or in order of priority.
   d. It is not necessary to separate the numbers in any way, so do not insert spaces, dashes, commas, slashes or any other spacing device between the numbers.

POINTS TO REMEMBER:
   Remember that there is only one correct sequence that preserves the client's safety at all stages during the procedure.

**GRAPHIC 13-2.
FILL-IN-THE-BLANK SEQUENCE ITEM**

Put the following words in alphabetical order.

1. Pizza
2. Apples
3. Onion
4. Bacon
5. Rice

Type your answer in the box below.

24315

Section III: Multiple Response

A. Overview
   1. Definition: Multiple response items are a type of alternate item that require you to choose more than one answer from up to six options. Any number of the options may be correct.
   2. Method of Answer: To answer these questions, you will need to click on all the answers that apply.
   3. On the NCLEX, you will receive credit only for completely correct answers; there is no "partial credit" given for these item types.

POINTS TO REMEMBER:

Consider each response as you would a true-false question; is that statement true about the question or false? Click on all that you determine are true.

GRAPHIC 13-3.
MULTIPLE RESPONSE ITEM

Which of the following are types of vegetables?

Select all that apply.

☑   1.   Broccoli

☑   2.   Cucumber

☐   3.   Peach

☐   4.   Orange

☐   5.   Grape

Section IV: Hot Spot

A. Overview
   1. Definition: Hot spot items are a type of alternate item that will be a "point and click" exercise. Hot spot items will usually require you to identify an anatomical location on a figure.
   2. Method of Answer: To answer these questions, you will need to point at an area on the screen with your cursor and click on the correct spot. As you move your mouse around the screen, you will see an arrow. Once you select a spot and click, the arrow will change into a circle with an "X" in it.
   3. Read the question carefully, then analyze the image.
   4. The NCLEX will allow you to reclick as many times as necessary.

POINTS TO REMEMBER:

It is very important to remember that the screen is NOT a mirror image! If you see that the question is asking for an answer on the right or left side of the body, make sure you are clicking on the correct side.

GRAPHIC 13-4.
HOT SPOT ITEM

The nurse is performing a cardiac assessment.
Identify where the nurse will place the stethoscope
to best auscultate the apical pulse.

Section V: Charts, Tables, & Graphic Images

A. Overview
1. Any of the NCLEX standard multiple choice or alternate items may also include charts, tables or other graphic images that you must analyze and understand in order to correctly answer the question.
2. It is important that you read the question carefully first, then analyze the image.

GRAPHIC 13-5.
CHARTS, TABLES, GRAPHIC IMAGES ITEM

This graph represents:

☑ 1. ECG
☐ 2. EEG
☐ 3. EMG
☐ 4. EGD

CD-ROM INSTALLATION INSTRUCTIONS

MEDS Publishing Software requires 50 MB of Hard Drive.

To install our software, apply the following steps:

1. Insert CD into CD-ROM drive.
2. Double click the My Computer icon
3. Double click the icon for your CD-ROM drive
4. Double click Setup.exe

NOTE:
Windows 2000 installation may receive an InstallShield dialog box "1207:Windows (R) Installer found." This is an older version of Windows (R) Installer. Click OK to Continue. Click OK.

3. Click the NEXT button to start the install and follow the on-screen instructions. A status bar displays the progress of the installation.
4. A window appears saying, "install complete."
   Click Finish.

To run MEDS' Software,

1. Go to Start, Programs, meds Software...
2. Locate and select the appropriate title.

You are ready to begin.